MILLY'S

— REAL FOOD —

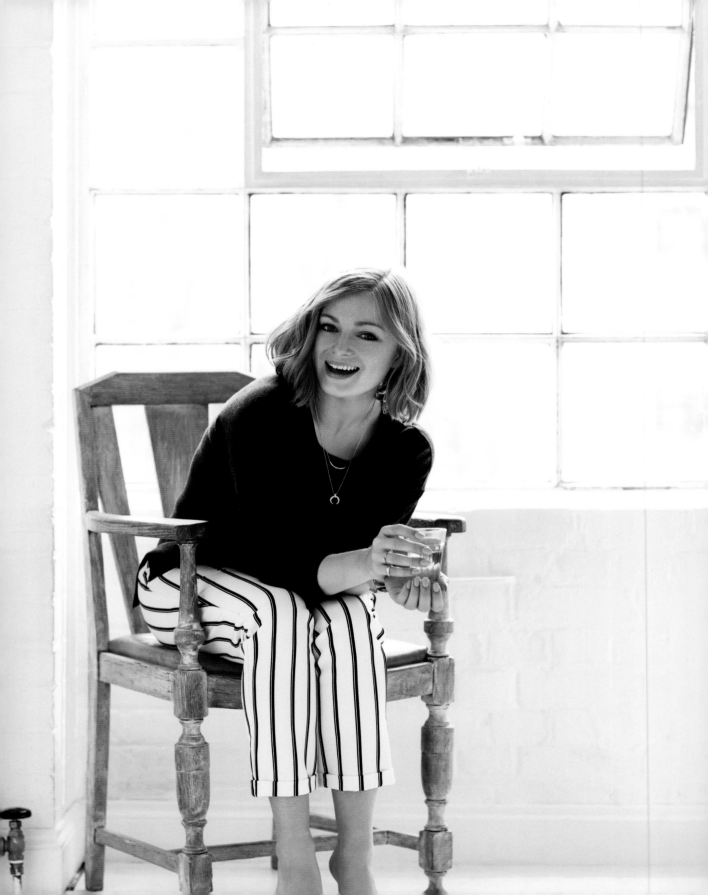

MILLY'S
— REAL FOOD —

NICOLA MILLBANK

HQ

For my Grandad, Walter, who at the ripe old age of 101 taught me
that "a little bit of what you fancy does you good."

HQ, an imprint of HarperCollins*Publishers*, 1 London Bridge Street, London, SE1 9GF

www.harpercollins.co.uk

First published by HQ, an imprint of HarperCollins*Publishers* 2017

Text © Nicola Millbank 2017

10 9 8 7 6 5 4 3 2 1

Nicola Millbank asserts the moral right to be identified as the author of this work

A catalogue record of this book is available from the British Library

ISBN 978-0-00-821503-3

Design: HQ | Louise McGrory
Editor: HQ | Rachel Kenny
Production: Milly Cookbook Ltd.
Photography: Susanna Blåvarg
Food stylist: Sara Assum Hultberg with Nicola Millbank
Props stylist: Susanna Blåvarg with Nicola Millbank
Clothing and jewellery: Missoma pp 6, 17, 150, 183, 185 and 189, Whistles p 52, COS Front cover and p 225, Cyberjammies p 45 and
Astley Clarke p 186
Make-up: Katie Nixon
Hair: Kieron Lavine
Recipe testing: Sara Assum Hultberg
Thank you also to Anthropology p 24, JJ Locations, The Culpeper and The Posh Burger Co.

Printed and bound in Spain

CONTENTS:

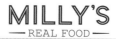

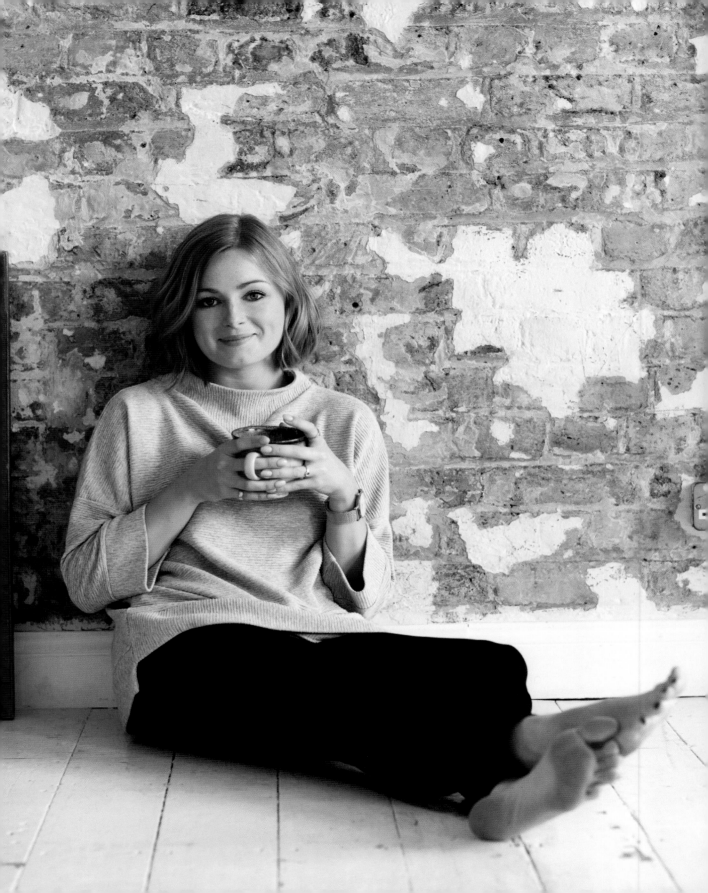

So, here we are.

If you're after a no-nonsense approach to home cooking, with a sprinkle of delicious recipes, a dash of reality and a ladle of EAT CARBS AND BE HAPPY, then this is your kind of book.

But before we go any further, a little bit about me. I'm an actress by trade, but I'm also a devoted foodie. And by that I mean I spend most of my spare time thinking up new recipes, writing about food, and dreaming about what I'm going to eat next. I live in London with my fiancé Mike and my miniature Dachshund Darcey, and in summer 2015 I set up a website, Milly Cookbook, to document my life in food. I had no idea then that my passion project would become a second all-consuming full-time job!

I don't do elimination diets. I do, however, eat just about everything, so don't be surprised if you see chicken wings or sweet potato gnocchi in here. My mantra is quite simple: Eat everything in moderation. So in this book you'll find recipes that embrace all ingredients and food groups from pancakes to paella, salads to sticky ribs.

Unless you've had your head in the sand, I'm sure you've heard of the "clean eating" trend that's been sweeping the nation. If that's your gig, then cool. As you were. But that's not my thing. My primary issue with the term "clean eating" is that it insinuates that unless you follow a sugar-free, alcohol-free (God forbid), gluten-free lifestyle, you are eating *dirty*. Eating a bowl of courgetti instead of spaghetti is about as appealing to me as eating a sponge. I do not get a kick out of that. And don't get me started with the raw-avocado-matcha-quinoa brownies . . . just have a brownie and enjoy it!

The worst thing for me, perhaps, is the term "guilt-free". In the early days, I toyed with this tagline, but it soon became very apparent that there was something fundamentally wrong with it and I asked myself the question, "Why do we need guilt-free alternatives?" This surely perpetuates the notion that we have something to feel guilty about. Why should we feel guilty for eating food that we enjoy? Why have we abandoned staples such as bread and pasta? "Enough of the self-persecuting, self-diagnosing and demonising food groups," I thought. "It's time to enjoy our food again."

Not an easy ideal to stick to when you're in my line of work, I'll admit. I'm privy to the pressures that are put on women (and men for that matter) to fit the narrow definition of what the media think a woman (or man) should look like. Although I love what I do, I can become impatient and frustrated with the industry. It's very fickle; judging people on their looks and not their talent. It could be very demoralising in the early days, but I quickly learnt that you have to grow a thick skin and just power through. It's important to be yourself and not succumb to the pressures put on everyone to look a certain way. I really look up to the women who defy these rules; who've turned their backs and called people out on it. They're the women who've made history.

Now, I know what some of you are thinking – an actress woke up one day, decided she wanted to do a book and so had an entire team of people writing it for her with her name slapped on the front, right? Wrong. Blood, sweat and tears have been poured into making this book, not only because I'm an utter control freak and wanted to be involved in every part of it, but because I was given the chance. My publisher took the rather brave step of handing over the creative reins, allowing me complete control over the photography, the food styling, the props – the whole look and feel of the book! And I think we've created something rather wonderful. I did a lot of research online before I stumbled upon a photographer – Susanna – whose work I loved, and I fired off an email with no expectations whatsoever. I was stunned when she emailed back to say she was available,

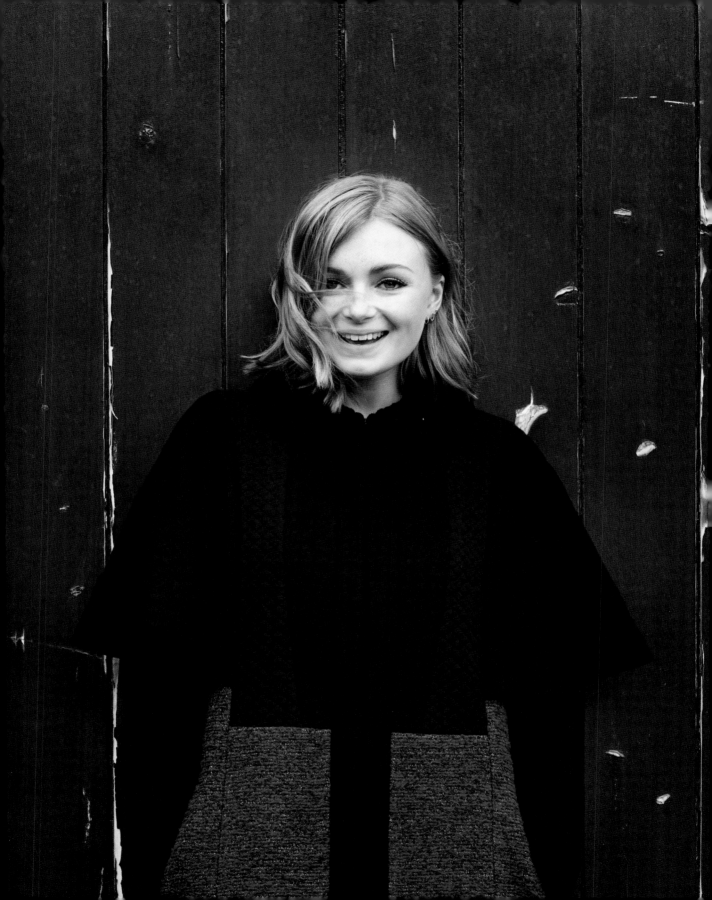

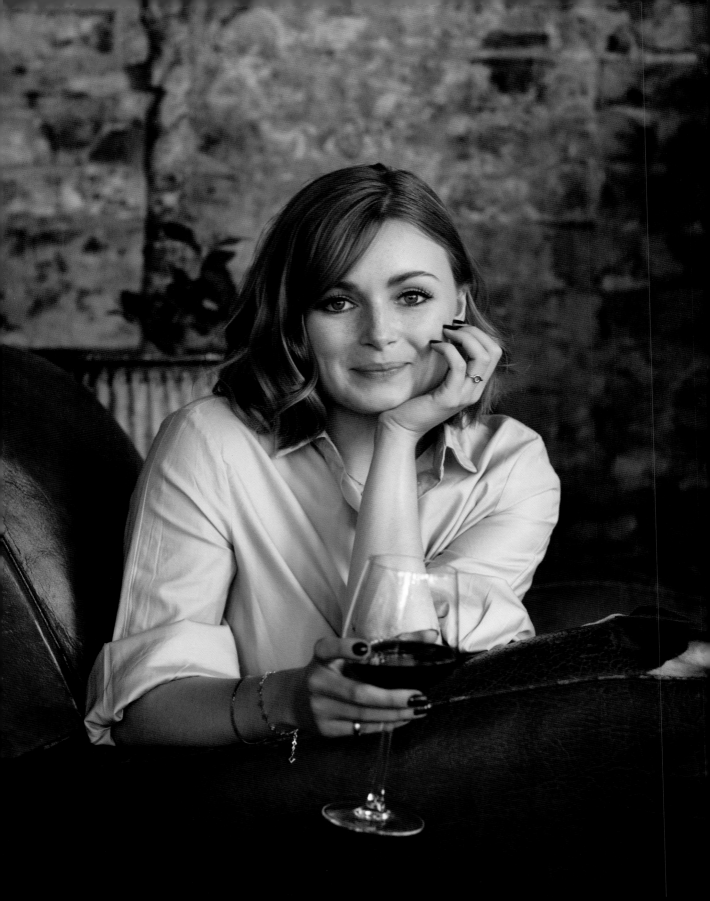

and she wanted to work with me! Next I found a beautiful and talented food stylist – Sara – and a team of fabulous hair and makeup artists and, we then shot the book in Stockholm, Sweden, returning to my distant Scandinavian roots to take inspiration from the colour schemes, the laidback attitude, effortlessly cool interiors and food. All of the recipes are mine: I've created them, tested them, tweaked them and now I want to share them with you. I've learnt so much already and I hope this is just the beginning of my food journey.

Growing up, I always sat down to dinner with my family. No matter what anyone was doing we always made it back to the table. The kitchen was the hub of our home; we cooked, we laughed, we cried, we ate and drank and caught up on the day's events together. Mealtimes equating togetherness is such an important mentality to have. Because of this I always associate food with family, talking and laughing – positivity. Snacking and eating on the go makes food become fuel. I'm very much a person who lives to eat and doesn't eat to live; it's such an important part of my life. Home cooking is, after all, what we all do. We survive on it every day. It is something we all have in common.

And this is why I want to celebrate the home cook again, dedicate my time to making real food and always aim for *lagom* (a Swedish term meaning "just the right amount").

When I moved to London aged 18, I started to try lots of new food from all over the world – from Japan to France via Portugal. My cooking, however, wasn't quite so cosmopolitan. Shepherd's Pie, stir-fries and tray bakes were pretty much all I could cook and I quickly tired of the beige monotony. Something had to change. Cooking became my hobby; I experimented with flavours, learnt a few of the basics and began curating dishes, many of which have made it into this book.

I'm not a chef – I never have been and I've never tried to be. (And, for the record,

I have appalling knife skills and I'm not afraid to admit it.) What I am, is passionate about home cooking, mixing flavours and experimenting with recipes that can be enjoyed with friends and family. Creating something that makes us happy and brings us all together.

So I wanted to create a book with recipes that were a fitting testament to that philosophy, using accessible and affordable ingredients – no weekly pay cheques spent at health food shops on coconut oil and spirulina. It's all about fresh, easy to find and reasonably priced produce, the best of British grub cooked to perfection and embracing Scandinavian, European, Mediterranean, Asian and Middle Eastern cuisines.

I also wanted to create a book that the generations of female cooks and chefs before me would be proud of. It's these ladies who have blazed a trail, and who have given me the courage to stand confidently by my values regarding what we eat, how we eat, and our relationship with food. This is my way of saying thank you to them. Above all, *Milly's Real Food* is a little bit of everything; how I like to eat at home and what I cook my friends and family. As my hero of a grandfather, Walter, would say: "A little bit of what you fancy does you good." Let's get cooking some *Real Food*.

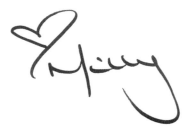

P.S. Share your recipe photos, favourite foodie haunts, meal ideas, and real food tips, tricks and hacks with me on Instagram @millycookbook or Twitter @MillyCookbook, with the hashtag #MillysRealFood

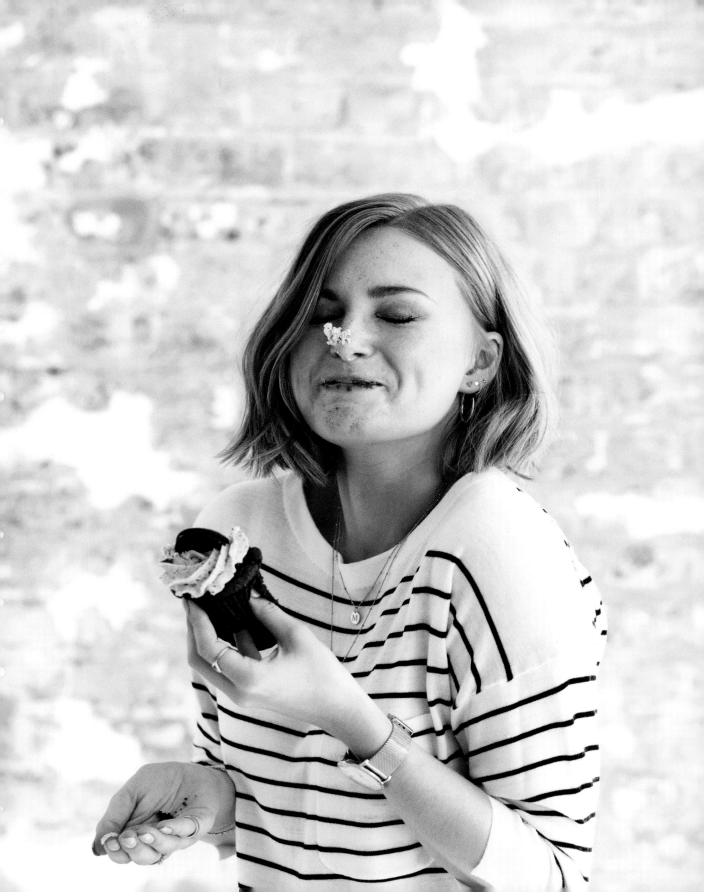

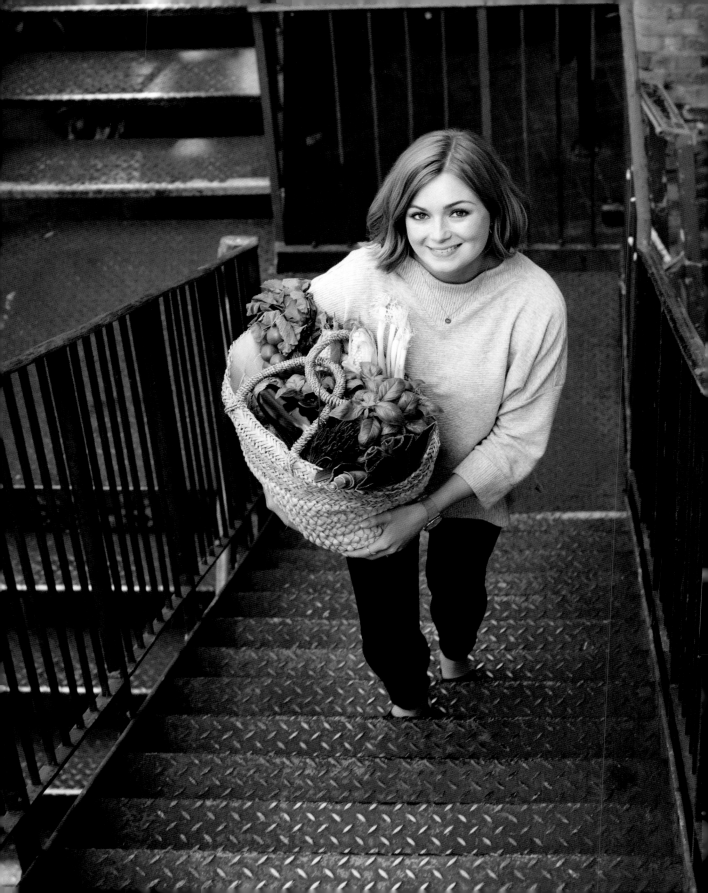

FRIDGE, FREEZER AND CUPBOARD ESSENTIALS

FRUIT & VEGETABLES

Berries: strawberries, blueberries and **raspberries** – perfect for breakfast, they can be frozen for smoothies and made into jams when they're on their way out. Lots of **lemons** and **limes** for easy seasoning and bringing a dish to life immediately. Anything green: **broccoli, green beans** and **sprouts** – fantastic sources of iron and easy to use as a base, just add a dressing or a sauce; grill or fry to make dinner a bit more exciting. **Mini Cos lettuce** and **cucumber** for their refreshing crunch, plus **celery, carrots** and **banana shallots** as the base for casseroles, ragu, pasta sauces and risotto.

DELI

Prosciutto or **Parma ham** – eat the slices as they are, or, for a twist, try frying them as a bacon alternative; add to stews and sauces for an extra kick of flavour. **Chorizo** – essential for Mike's Paella (p 112) and a game-changer with seared scallops and in chicken dishes.

DAIRY

Halloumi and **feta** cheese and the full-on **stinky blues.** Full fat, salted **butter.** **Parmesan** to make any savoury dish sing, and it lasts forever.

MEAT

Chicken – buy a whole bird, roast it and live off the leftovers for days: cost-effective and extremely versatile. **Beef brisket, chuck** and **oxtail** for slow-cooked and hearty ragu. **Pork** or **beef mince** for Bolognese: double up the ingredients and you can freeze portions for later meals. Good-quality **sausages** have more uses than just bangers and mash: squeeze the meat out into pasta sauces and slice them into stews.

FISH

Salmon, cod and **prawns** – quick to cook, packed full of goodness and easy to rustle up a meal in minutes.

WHAT TO KEEP IN YOUR CUPBOARD

VEGETABLES

Potatoes – sweet potatoes, new potatoes and Desirée for the best dauphinoise. **Mushrooms**: chestnut, shiitake, enoki, oyster – the weirder, the better. Do try different ones. **Tomatoes** in all shapes and colours, if you can find them – perfect as a light lunch with mozzarella and a staple for homemade tomato sauce.

OILS

Extra-virgin olive oil – the best you can afford, for drizzling. **Rapeseed oil** for cooking because it has a higher smoke point, which means it retains its nutritional qualities even after being heated. **Toasted sesame oil** makes Asian dishes really wonderful.

HERBS & SPICES

Chilli flakes, dried rosemary, thyme and **oregano** are my cupboard essentials and go into so many of my recipes. **Chinese five spice, curry powder** and **turmeric** lend themselves to lots of dishes, adding colour and a delicious depth of flavour. Ground and whole **cinnamon** works brilliantly in savoury and sweet dishes and drinks. **Saffron** is, without doubt, the most decadent, but a little goes a long way. Add to the cooking water when preparing rice for a fragrant dish or work into seafood pasta sauces. Salt *must* be **flaked sea salt.** Don't bother with table salt to season your food, leave that for the pasta water.

BREAD & BISCUITS

ANYTHING – I'm pro-carbs. **Pitta, bagels, tortillas, fluffy white loaf, crackers** and **oatcakes** are my favourites and form the basis of an instant delicious lunch or substantial snack (there's no beating a ham and cheese toastie when you're starving and the cupboard is bare). Store bread in the freezer if you don't manage to get through a whole loaf or pack in 3 days.

WHAT TO KEEP IN YOUR CUPBOARD

EGGS

Free-range hen's eggs (also **duck eggs** are tasty and available at a lot of big supermarkets).

CONDIMENTS

Stock jelly or cubes save dishes which need that extra oomph; **soy sauce, oyster sauce, Sriracha** (the only hot sauce worth its salt) and **hoisin** are all essential for Asian dishes; **peanut butter** – dollop into sauces and dips, fry with chicken and add to noodles and broth for an extra kick; **Marmite** – treat it like stock in stews and ragu, it adds a different element to a hearty dish; **wholegrain and Dijon mustard** work their way into almost every vegetable side dish of mine as well as salad dressings.

DRIED & GRAINS

Pasta: Love it all, but **lasagne sheets** are my cupboard essential. **White and brown rice, Arborio risotto rice** and **pearl barley** – different but my absolute favourite and pleasingly chewy.

TINNED

I always have jars of **passata** and tins of **tomatoes** – cherry, chopped or whole. They go into every Italian pasta dish and stew – I buy them by the truck-load. **Coconut cream** is much better than coconut milk, it has ten times more flavour. **Chickpeas** – a single tin of chickpeas can make a tub of homemade hummus; I also like to roast them and drench with hot sauce to make a tasty snack.

WHAT TO PUT IN YOUR FREEZER

PASTA & PASTRY

Fresh **ravioli, tagliatelle** and **spaghetti**, **wanton wrappers**; **puff, filo** and **shortcrust pastry** all live in my freezer. Cook the pasta from frozen and thaw pastry for a couple of hours before needed.

MEAT & FISH

Everything is fine in the freezer, but do double-check how long you can keep your meat and fish in there before using it. Look out for freezer bags of **prawns** – I love these. Take as many out as you want and it's much cheaper than buying fresh every time.

READY-TO-GO

We all have nights when taking a meal from the freezer and heating it through, then snuggling down in front of the TV, is the only viable option. For those days, my go-to ready-made meals are prepared dim sum (which survive the trip from freezer to plate much better than you would expect), gnocchi, soup and pre-prepared gravy in zipper bags, cooked Bolognese and portioned lasagne, stew and ragu ready to heat up. Every time I make a dish, I make double.

ICE CREAM

PLENTY OF IT.

A NOTE ON MEAT, FISH, EGGS AND DAIRY

If I can be pushy on any point, it is here. Please, please buy British farm-assured free-range and organic meat, eggs and dairy and responsibly sourced fish. Although our country has a high standard of animal welfare, sometimes things fall through the cracks of system. It can cost more, but it doesn't have to be a lot more – especially if you plan your meals and use cheaper cuts of meat, such as chicken thighs or wings, beef chuck and oxtail.

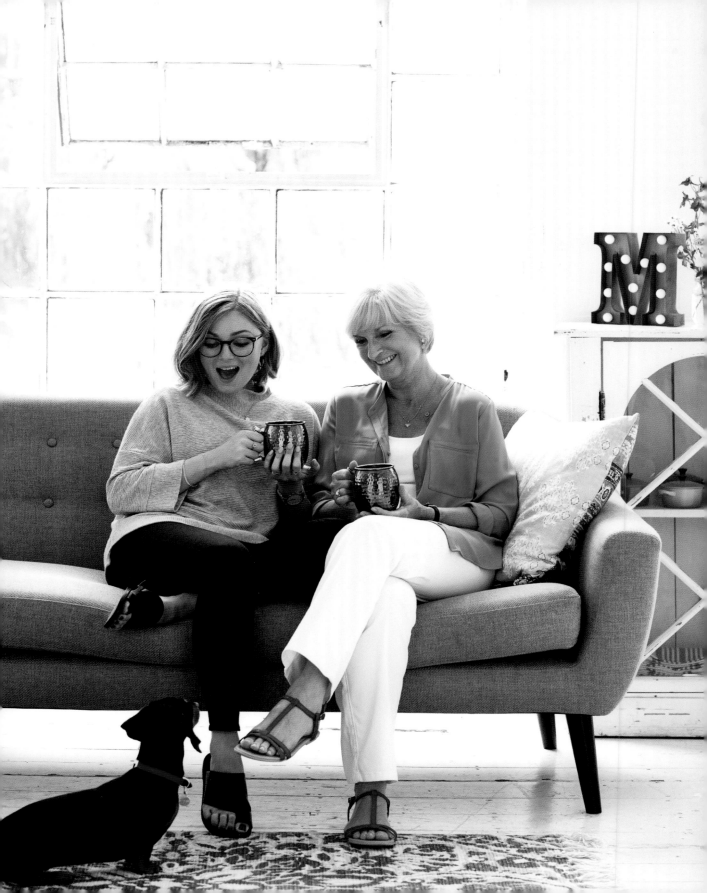

BRUNCH

"One should not attend even the end of the world without a good breakfast."
Robert A. Heinlein

Undoubtedly, my favourite meal of the day. Even saying it fills me with happiness. Creamy eggs Benedict, smoked salmon, Shakshuka (a Middle Eastern dish of eggs in a spicy tomato sauce), endless cups of coffee, Bloody Marys and smoothies – at home or out with friends. No one is happier than I am that brunch has become part of our culture, with British restaurants and cafés putting it centre stage, and priding themselves on their carefully considered brunch-centric menus.

Admittedly, it's not just the food aspect of brunch that I love – it's what it represents. For me, it means the weekend hustle and bustle of friends, families and loved ones in the village-like part of town where I live, clumps of people sitting in the sunshine nursing a hangover, or tucking into a large bacon sandwich washed down with two cappuccinos.

I am even eating brunch as I write this chapter. Darcey is curled up next to me, and I couldn't be happier.

In this chapter I've included the dishes I like to make for myself throughout the week, for friends on Saturdays, and for Mike and me on a lazy Sunday morning. From pancakes to popsicles, frittatas to fritters, there's something for everyone.

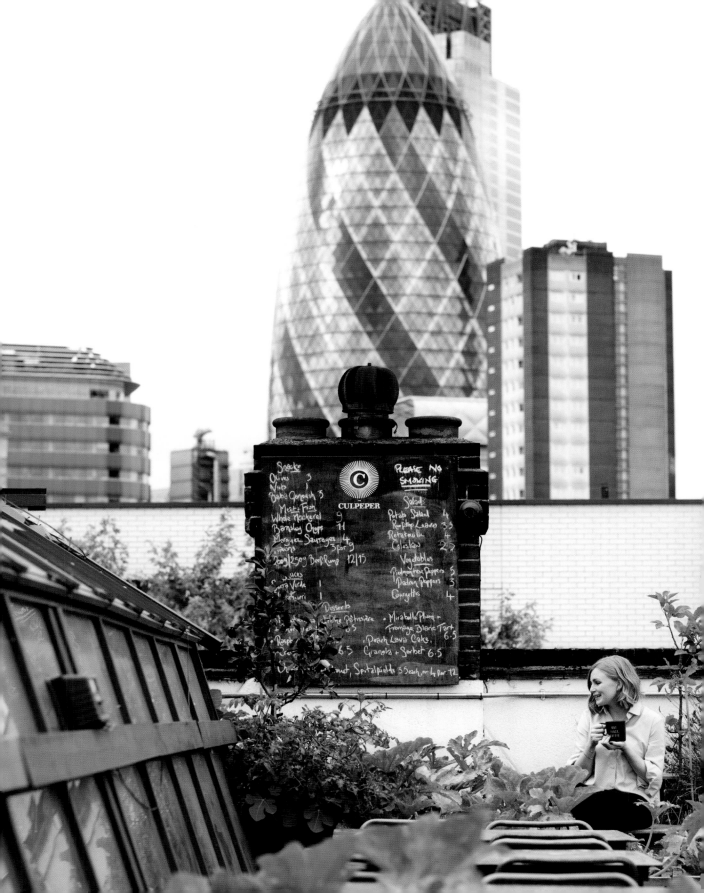

JUICES AND SMOOTHIES

SERVES
2

There's something seriously refreshing and satisfying about juices and smoothies. If I'm feeling a little over-indulged, a juice first thing sorts me out and makes me feel a bit better. It's also a brilliant snack or a super breakfast on the run if you're in a hurry. These are, however, not designed to be regular meal-replacers but rather an extra element to your breakfast. Have one alongside your pancakes or frittata!

MILLY GREEN JUICE

INGREDIENTS :

2 green apples
1 pear
2 celery sticks
½ lime, peeled
½ cucumber
a large handful of spinach
100ml coconut water or
tap water

METHOD :

Pop everything through a juicer and serve over ice. If you don't have a juicer, blend in a food processor or smoothie maker and pass through a sieve over a bowl.

APPLE, ORANGE, CARROT AND GINGER JUICE

INGREDIENTS :

6 carrots
3 apples
1 orange, peeled
½ lemon, peeled
a thumb-sized piece of
ginger, peeled

METHOD :

Put all your ingredients through a juicer and serve over ice. If you don't have a juicer, blend in a processor or smoothie maker and pass through a sieve over a bowl.

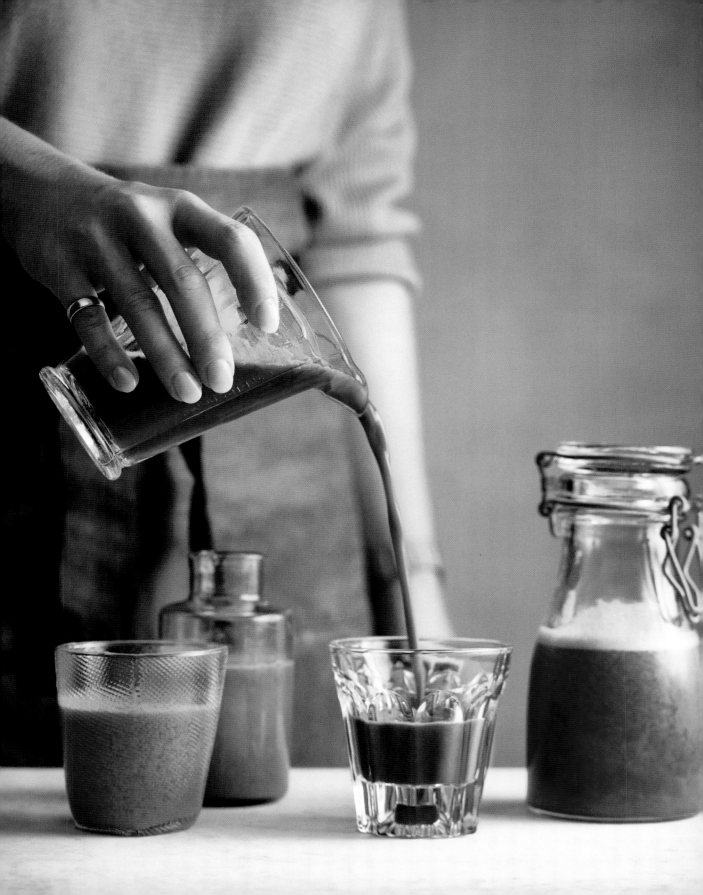

JUICES AND SMOOTHIES
CONT...

SERVES
2

PINK LEMONADE

INGREDIENTS:

1 pink grapefruit, peeled
2 Pink Lady apples or any sweet
apple variety
a handful of fresh raspberries,
plus extra to garnish
100ml sparkling water
honey, to taste
a sprig of fresh mint

METHOD:

Pop the grapefruit, apple and most of the raspberries in a juicer.
If you don't have a juicer, blend in a processor or smoothie
maker and pass through a sieve over a bowl.
  Pour in the sparkling water, add honey to taste and if you'd
like, serve over ice with a couple of fresh raspberries and sprig
of mint.

PINEAPPLE, CUCUMBER AND MINT JUICE

INGREDIENTS:

½ pineapple
1 cucumber
1 large handful of mint,
stalks removed
a thumb-sized piece of
ginger, peeled

METHOD:

Pop everything through a juicer and serve over ice. If you don't
have a juicer, blend in a processor or smoothie maker and pass
through a sieve over a bowl.

SERVES
2

CHOCOLATE PEANUT BUTTER SMOOTHIE

INGREDIENTS:

2 bananas
1 tbsp cocoa powder
1 tbsp crunchy peanut butter
200ml skimmed milk
honey, to taste

METHOD:

Blitz the first 4 ingredients in a smoothie maker or blender, adding honey to taste. The sweetness of the smoothie will depend on how ripe your bananas are.

BANANA, DATE AND CINNAMON SMOOTHIE

INGREDIENTS:

2 bananas
6 Medjool dates
2 tsp cinnamon
200ml skimmed milk

METHOD:

Blitz all the ingredients in a smoothie maker or blender and serve immediately.

COURGETTE, ASPARAGUS AND FETA EGG WHITE FRITTATA

This one's for gym bunnies. As most of us know, egg whites are absolutely packed with protein and good to eat after a morning workout. However, this frittata is way more exciting. Fresh asparagus, courgette, basil and a good sprinkling of salty, crumbly feta make for a very tasty but healthy breakfast.

INGREDIENTS:

olive oil, for brushing
8 egg whites, beaten
100g feta
1 small courgette, cut
into ribbons
3–4 asparagus spears, thinly
sliced at an angle
sea salt and freshly ground
black pepper

TO SERVE:

fresh basil leaves
extra-virgin olive oil,
for drizzling

TIP:

For a more economical approach, look out for cartons of egg whites in your supermarket. You will need about half a carton, as there are usually 15 egg whites in a carton.

METHOD:

Preheat the oven to 180°C/160°C fan/Gas mark 4.

Pop the pan over a medium–high heat, lightly brush with olive oil and pour in the egg whites. Season with a good pinch of salt and pepper.

Crumble in half the feta and add the courgette and asparagus. Mix gently and then stick in the oven for 20 minutes until cooked and the top is starting to brown. Allow to stand for a few minutes.

To serve, slide the frittata out of the pan and place on a plate, then top with the rest of the feta, some fresh basil leaves and a drizzle of extra-virgin olive oil.

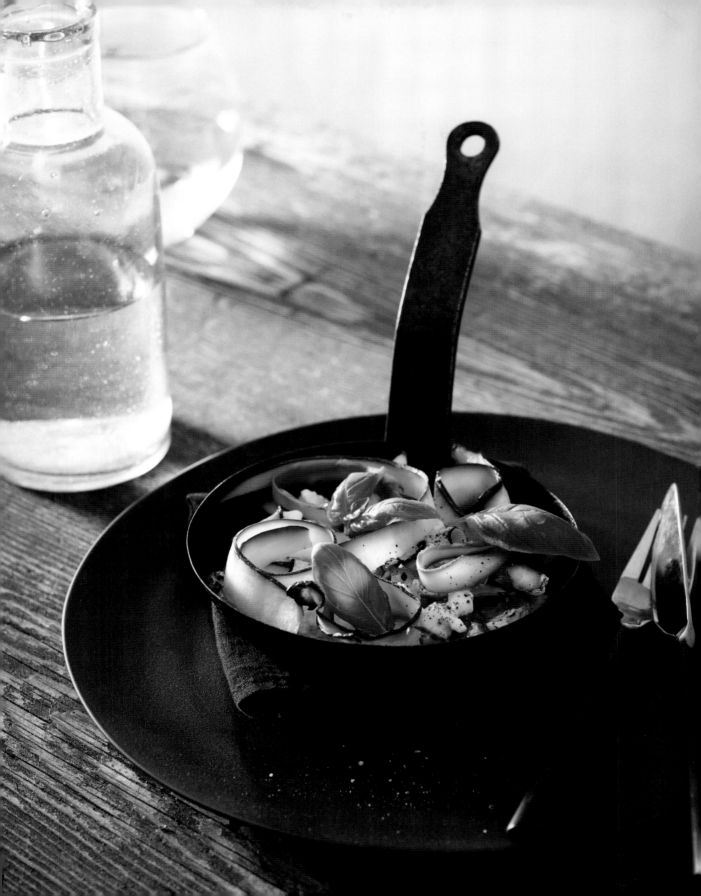

GREEK BAKED EGGS

This is one of my all-time favourite brunch dishes. A Greek take on the classic spicy tomato sauce and poached egg dish Shakshuka, with fresh herbs, tangy feta and salty olives. It's really simple to make; just have all of your ingredients ready and a big doorstop wedge of bread to mop it all up with. And as we're among friends, this is pretty darn good for the day after the night before.

INGREDIENTS:

olive oil
½ medium onion,
finely chopped
1 garlic clove, finely chopped
1 tsp dried sage
1 tsp dried oregano
1 tsp dried rosemary
1 x 400g tin chopped tomatoes
1 tsp sugar
4–5 fresh cherry
tomatoes, halved
a handful of pitted black olives,
halved
100g fresh feta, crumbled
2 eggs
sea salt and freshly ground
black pepper

TO SERVE:

a few sprigs of fresh herbs
(oregano, thyme or basil), chopped
a thick wedge of bread

METHOD:

Heat a glug of olive oil in a small frying pan over a medium heat. Add the onion and fry for a few minutes until soft, then add the garlic, sage, oregano and rosemary and cook for 1 minute.

Add the tinned tomatoes and bring to a simmer. Add the sugar, a pinch of salt and pepper and leave to simmer for 5–7 minutes until the sauce has reduced.

Add the fresh tomatoes, olives and half the feta to the pan and stir well.

Make two wells in the tomato mixture and crack in the eggs. If your pan is ovenproof, pop under a hot grill for 5–10 minutes (depending on how runny you like your yolk) or simply place a lid on the pan and steam-cook the eggs.

Scatter with the fresh herbs, the remaining feta and a drizzle of extra-virgin olive oil, then dig in with a wedge of bread.

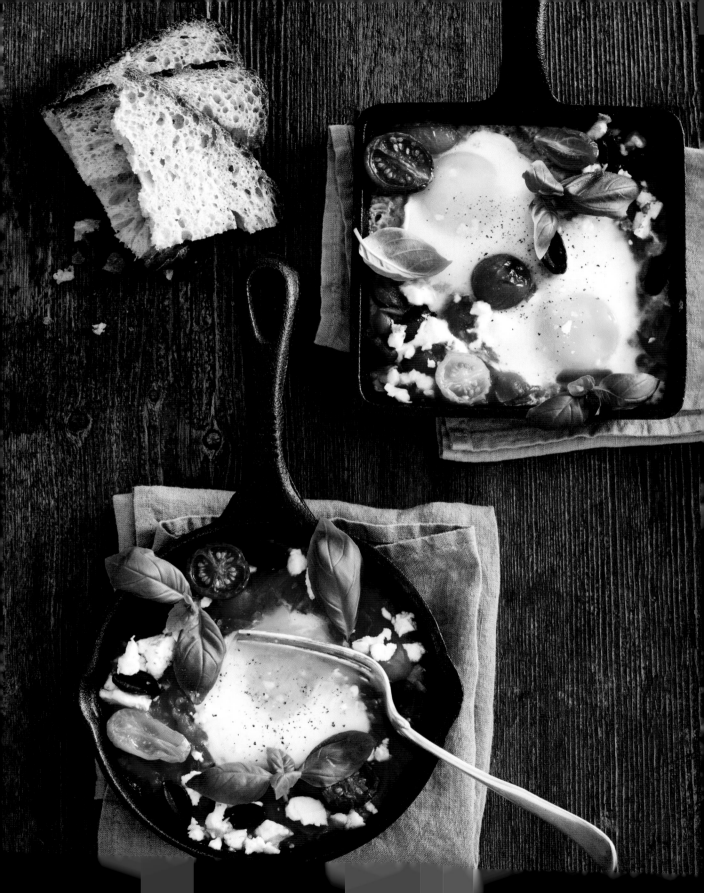

CASHEW, CRANBERRY AND COCONUT GRANOLA

MAKES
1 jar

I often make this granola recipe for Christmas. I'll make a big batch, stuff it into a mason jar, and tie a bow around it. It's so simple to make, not only a fantastic gift but really rather tasty. If you can't get hold of cranberries, raisins will work just as well. I'm not a big fan of coconut oil (in cooking anyway), but for this it really adds to the flavour. If, however, you can't get hold of any or don't want to spend the money on a whole jar (I don't blame you), then groundnut oil is a good substitute.

INGREDIENTS:

2 mugs rolled oats

1 mug dried cranberries

1 mug cashew nuts

½ mug sunflower seeds

2 tbsp desiccated coconut

3 tbsp honey

1 tbsp melted coconut oil /or groundnut oil

METHOD:

Preheat the oven to 160°C/150°C fan/Gas mark 3.

In a large bowl, add the oats, cranberries, cashews, sunflower seeds and desiccated coconut and stir well until everything is combined.

Line a baking tray with baking parchment. Add the honey and coconut or groundnut oil to the bowl. Stir well so the oats are fully coated, then spread out on the baking sheet.

Bake in the oven for 10 minutes, then remove and give it a good mix up, before returning to the oven for a further 10 minutes. Keep an eye on it in case it starts to burn.

Once golden, remove from the oven and allow to cool completely before putting in an airtight container. The granola will keep for up to 2 weeks.

CINNAMON HAZELNUT MILK

MAKES
1 litre

This will surprise you. I know it sounds a bit weird. Why would you make hazelnut milk when there's a pint of regular milk in the fridge? I get you. But have you ever felt a bit "claggy" after eating or drinking too much dairy? Or do you sometimes just fancy something a bit different? My cinnamon hazelnut milk is so easy to make, it's nuts… It works really well with Cashew, Cranberry and Coconut Granola (opposite) or even better in a hot chocolate.

INGREDIENTS:

1 mug raw hazelnuts
1 tsp vanilla paste or extract
1 tsp cinnamon
1 tbsp honey, optional

METHOD:

Place the hazelnuts, vanilla, cinnamon, honey and 900ml water in a jar or a covered bowl, give it a good stir and leave to soak overnight.

The next day, pop the entire mixture in a blender and blend until smooth.

Place some muslin or a very clean tea towel over another bowl. Pour the hazelnut and water mix into the centre of the tea towel sitting in the bowl, and carefully gather up the edges to create a ball-shaped pouch. Squeeze as much of the hazelnut milk out into the bowl as you can and then pour into a jar and keep in the fridge. It will keep for a few days.

LIGHT BANANA PANCAKES
WITH ORANGE DRIZZLE

SERVES
2

I must have been American in a previous life because to me, there is no better thing than pancakes and bacon with lashings of maple syrup. Ever the optimist, I like to think eating this on a frequent basis won't do too much damage, but I think we all know where that discussion is heading (after all, it's a little bit of what you fancy that'll do you good, not plate after plate!). Instead, on the days I have a pancake craving, I make these. Banana is mashed into the batter so you don't need to use as much flour and you get a light and airy batter that cooks just as well.

INGREDIENTS:

2 ripe bananas
2 eggs
4 level tbsp self-raising flour
2 tsp vegetable oil, for brushing
6 tbsp icing sugar
zest and juice of 1 orange

TO SERVE:

a handful of fresh raspberries

METHOD:

In a blender, blitz the bananas, eggs and flour until smooth. Allow the mixture to rest for a few minutes.

Heat a non-stick pan over a medium heat and brush with the vegetable oil. Ladle tennis ball-sized dollops onto the pan and cook for a couple of minutes until bubbles form on the surface – now they are ready to flip. Using a spatula or fish slice, carefully flip each pancake over one by one.

Cook the pancakes for another minute or two, then transfer onto kitchen paper. You may need to cook the pancakes in batches of 3–4 depending on the size of your pan.

Mix the icing sugar with enough orange juice and zest to form a loose icing with a drizzling consistency. Stack the pancakes, drizzle with the orange icing and serve with fresh raspberries.

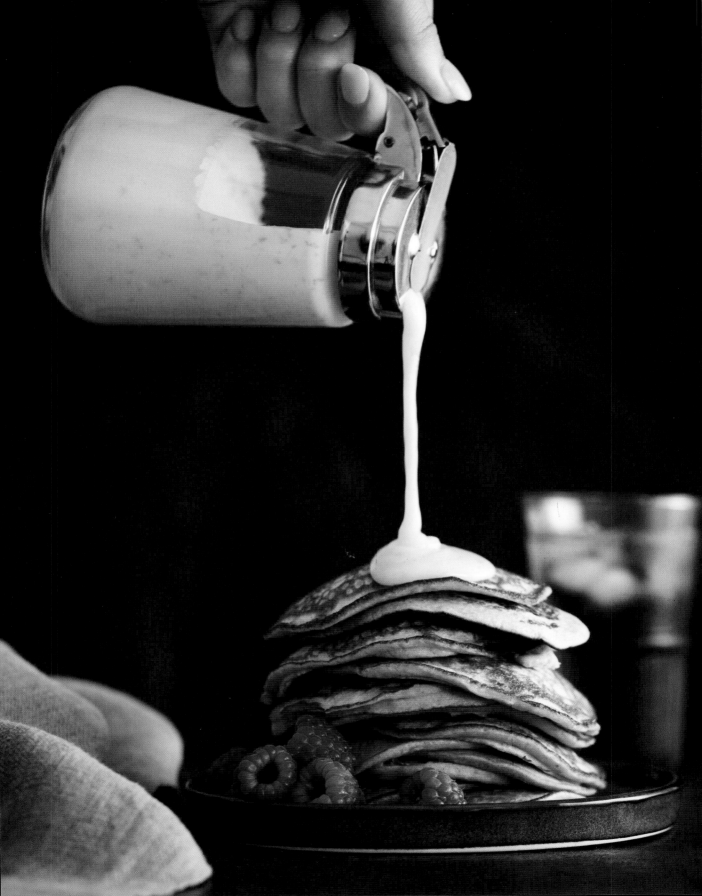

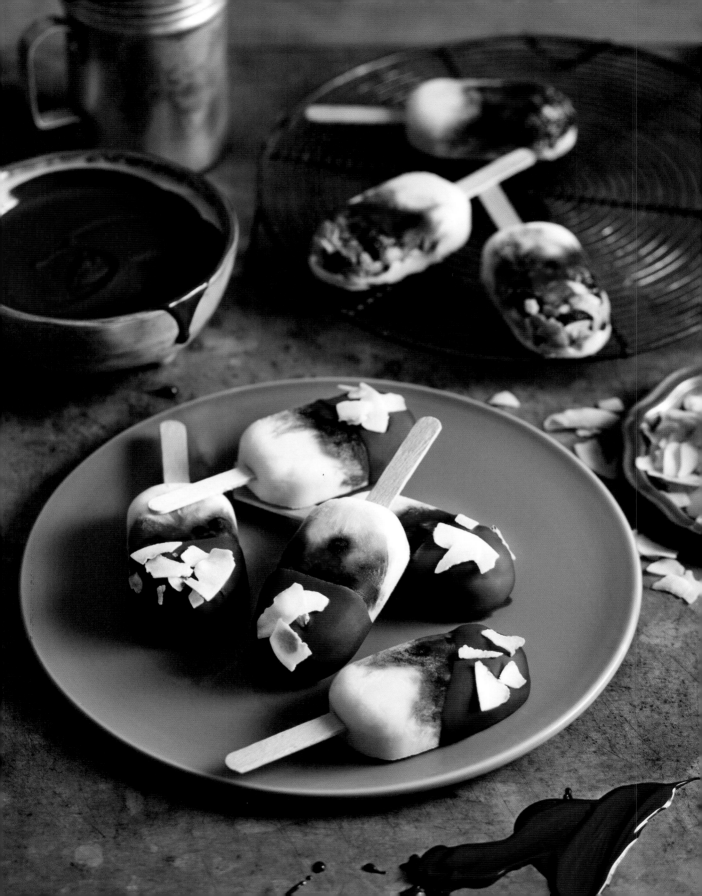

BERRY AND GRANOLA FROZEN YOGHURT LOLLIES

SERVES
4

Granola, berries and Greek yoghurt in a lolly? Oh yes. You can thank me later for this one, because it will be very popular with kids and adults alike. You can switch up what you put into them – try grated apple or a natural fruit yoghurt, if you fancy. These feel like a treat but they're actually a healthy breakfast.

INGREDIENTS:

4 tbsp mixed frozen berries
4 tbsp granola (try my Cashew, Cranberry and Coconut Granola, page 38)
2 tbsp honey
4 tbsp Greek yoghurt
2 tbsp melted dark chocolate, optional

METHOD:

Remove the berries from the freezer and allow to thaw slightly.

Mix together the granola and honey and press into the bottom of the ice lolly moulds.

Add a tablespoon of frozen berries and press down, then spoon over the Greek yoghurt to fill the mould.

Insert the lolly sticks and freeze for 3–4 hours or overnight.

If you want to make them that bit more decadent, dip the lollies in melted chocolate and freeze again before serving.

EQUIPMENT:

4 ice lolly moulds and sticks

MUM'S TOASTED LEMON DRIZZLE AGAVE BREAD

My mum is my hero, my best friend and the best lemon sultana loaf maker. This recipe is a corker and delicious served in slices with afternoon tea. My favourite way to eat it, however, is when it's a few days old. Simply toast a slice and spread with butter or my Lemon, Lime and Thyme Curd recipe on page 210.

Lemon, Lime and Thyme Curd recipe on page 210.

MAKES
1 loaf

INGREDIENTS:

225g golden sultanas
1 tsp bicarbonate of soda
225g self-raising flour
100g very cold butter, cubed
juice and zest of 1
unwaxed lemon
100g agave syrup
1 egg, beaten
sea salt

EQUIPMENT:

2lb (900g) loaf tin, greased and lined with greaseproof paper

TIP:

If you don't have agave syrup, that's no problem. Just use honey instead.

METHOD:

Preheat the oven to 170°C/150°C fan/Gas mark 3.

Put the sultanas into a bowl with 150ml boiling water and stir in the bicarbonate of soda. Set aside to cool.

In a large bowl, sift the flour and a pinch of salt, and rub in the butter until it resembles fine breadcrumbs, then add the lemon zest.

With a metal spoon, stir in the agave syrup, lemon juice, egg, sultanas and their soaking liquid. Gently fold everything together until combined.

Pour into the prepared tin and bake in the middle of the oven for 40–50 minutes or until the top is golden and an inserted skewer comes out clean.

Allow to cool fully on a wire rack before slicing.

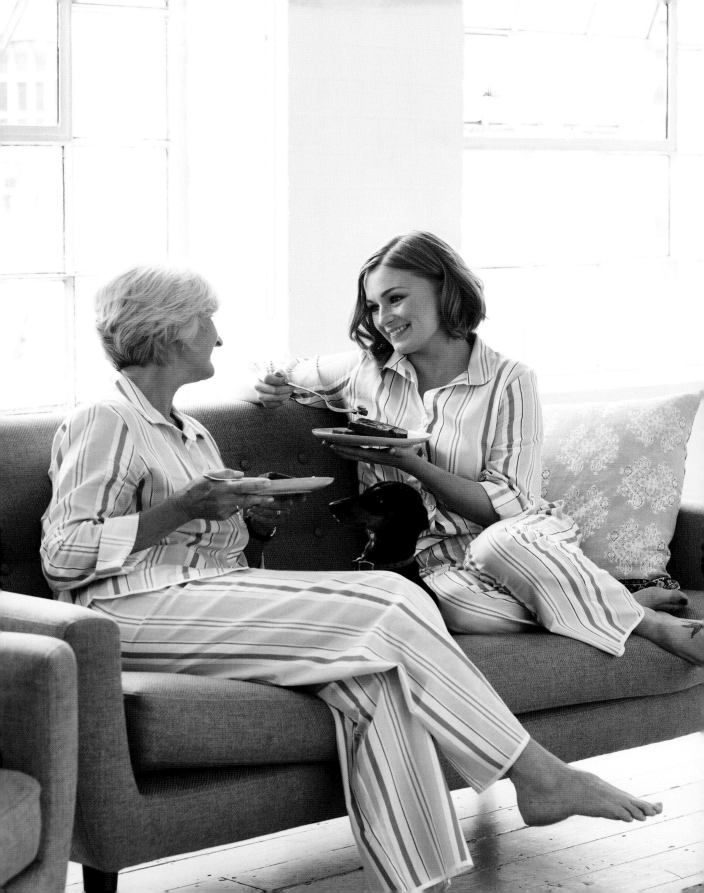

HALLOUMI, PROSCIUTTO AND SMASHED AVOCADO SARNIE
WITH MUSTARD MAPLE SYRUP DIP

SERVES
2

There's something immensely satisfying about dipping a sandwich into maple syrup, and when the sandwich contains everything you want from a breakfast sarnie, you're onto a winner. This is the best possible combination of salty and sweet, tangy and mellow. If you don't like avocado, replace with fresh spinach or sliced tomatoes and dip away.

INGREDIENTS:

2 tsp olive oil
250g halloumi cheese, sliced into 6 slices
90g prosciutto, about 6 slices
a small loaf of artisan crusty bread, such as sourdough
1 avocado
100ml maple syrup
1 tsp mustard seeds
2 tsp olive oil

METHOD:

Heat the olive oil in a non-stick pan over a medium–high heat. Add the halloumi slices and cook for 1–2 minutes on each side until golden brown. Transfer to a plate lined with kitchen paper and set aside.

Add the prosciutto slices to the same pan and cook for a few minutes until crisp. Transfer to the same plate as the halloumi.

Pop the slices of bread down into the pan and toast for a couple of minutes on each side until slightly charred.

Slice the avocado in half, remove the stone and spoon the flesh into a bowl. Using a fork, mash the avocado until it has a chunky consistency.

To assemble the sandwiches, spread one side of the toasted bread with half the avocado mixture, top with halloumi and prosciutto and top with the other piece of bread. Repeat.

Split the maple syrup between two mini bowls with half a teaspoon of mustard seeds in each. Simply dunk the sarnies in the mustard maple syrup for a pop of sweet and heat!

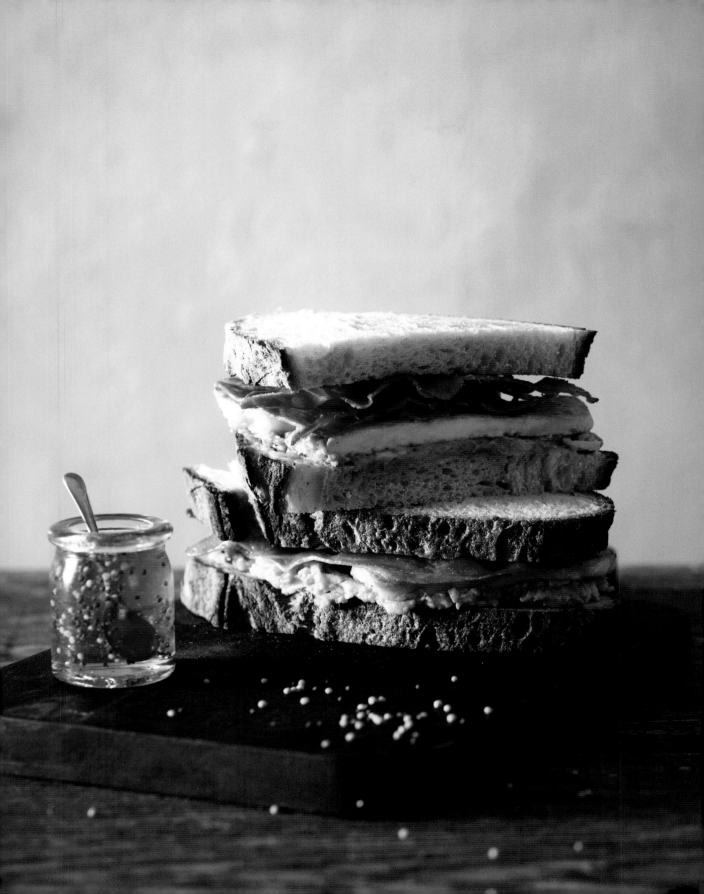

SWEETCORN FRITTERS,
WITH BACON AND A QUICK TOMATO CHUTNEY

SERVES
4
CHUTNEY MAKES
1 MEDIUM-SIZED JAR

Deep-fried fritters and bacon for breakfast – YES! This dish is my go-to for Sunday brunch, and whenever I make it I'm left with a delicious jar of tomato chutney in the fridge to have with cheese and biscuits later. This is a light batter, so the sweetcorn doesn't get eclipsed and the fritter's not too doughy.

INGREDIENTS:

FOR THE CHUTNEY:

200g red onion, finely chopped
400g tomatoes, deseeded and
roughly chopped
60ml red wine vinegar
120g brown sugar
1 tsp dried oregano
sea salt and freshly ground
black pepper

FOR THE FRITTERS:

2 eggs
2 banana shallots, peeled
and cut into rings
1 x 198g tin sweetcorn,
drained
120g plain flour
1 tsp chilli flakes
1 tsp paprika
1 tbsp vegetable oil
8 rashers streaky bacon
sea salt and freshly ground
black pepper

METHOD:

To make the chutney, place all the ingredients in a pan over a medium heat. Season with a good pinch of salt and pepper and stir well to combine. Simmer for 30–40 minutes or until it's reduced and sticky. Pour into a sterilised jar and allow to cool. This will keep for up to 4 weeks in the fridge.

To make the fritters, combine the eggs, shallots and sweetcorn, then add the flour, chilli flakes, paprika and seasoning.

Heat the vegetable oil in a non-stick pan over a medium heat. To test if the oil is hot enough, drop a little of the batter into the pan; it should start to sizzle straight away.

Using two teaspoons, spoon the batter into the pan and fry for a couple of minutes on each side until golden brown. Remove from the pan and drain on kitchen paper. Depending on the size of your pan you may need to cook the fritters in batches.

Fry the bacon in the same pan until crisp, then remove and drain on kitchen paper.

Serve the fritters with bacon and a good dollop of tomato chutney.

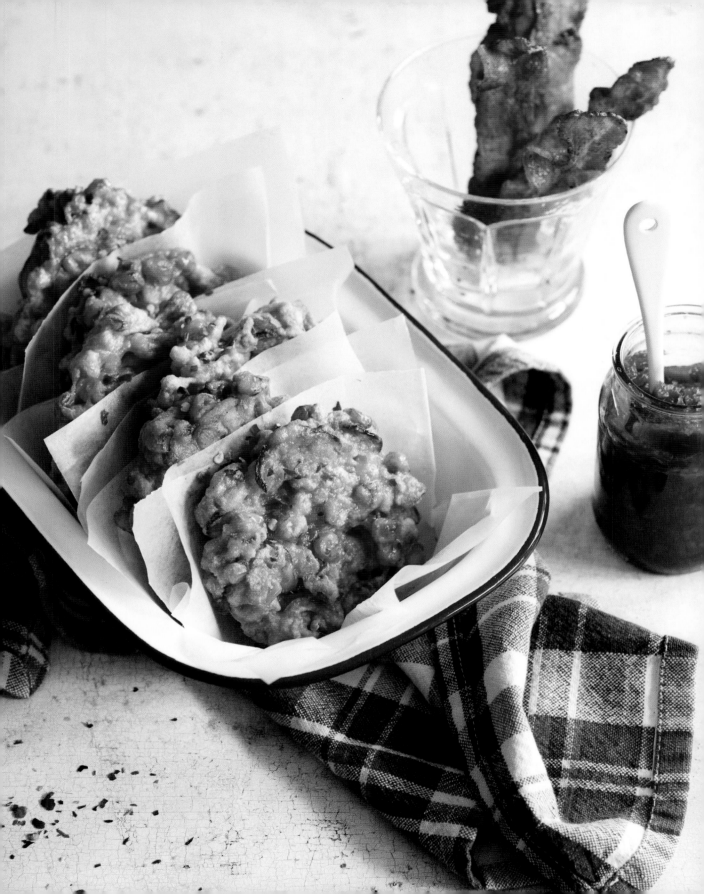

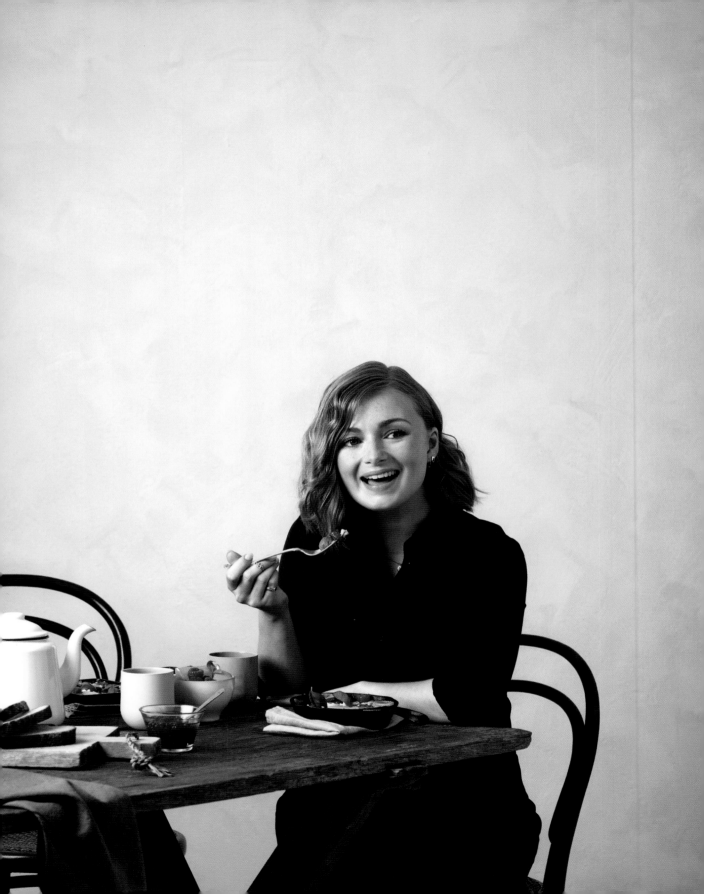

GIRLS' BRUNCH

What better way to get your friends over than to host brunch? For me, this is the ultimate Girls' Brunch. Prosecco at the ready! If you make the loaf, curd and lollies the day before, you can easily throw the rest of this together on a Sunday morning – it's just a case of making the potato cakes and whizzing up your drinks.

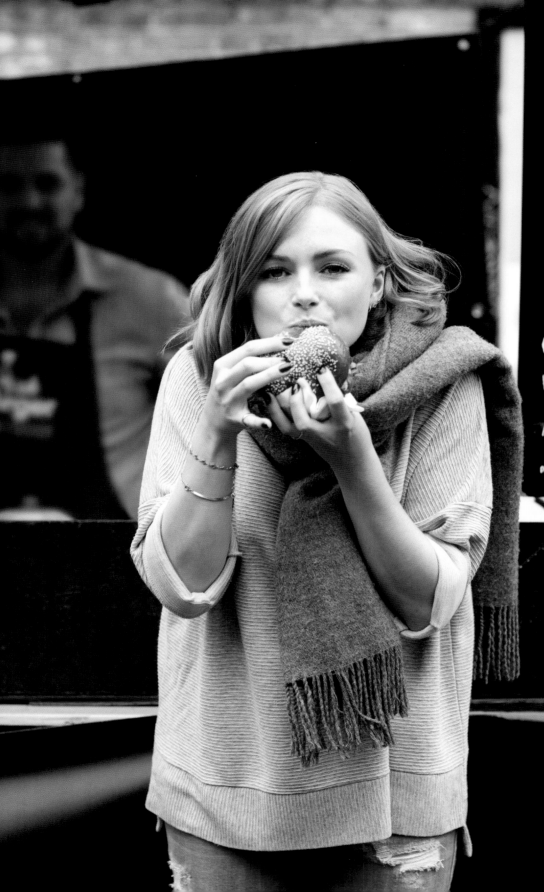

POSH CHEE

28 Day Dry Aged Steak P
Fresh Rocket, Caramelised

POSH CHEE

28 Day Dry Aged Steak
or Blue Cheese, Smokey May

POSH B*ST

Posh Cheese but with

CHIPS COOKE

Hand cut Maris Piper potato

All Burgers cooked to medium

PLEASE ADVISE US IF YOU HAV   ANY ALLERG

LIGHT BITES

"If you're afraid of butter, use cream."
Julia Child

LIGHT BITES

This chapter is all about two things: lunch and small plates. Dishes to be shared, or smaller-sized meals when you're peckish. Often, if I've been out during the day, I won't want a large meal for dinner, so instead I'll make something small or a "light bite".

Aside from our inherited brunch culture, I like to think us Brits also love to have a little bit of everything. I certainly do, and when I meet my mum for lunch this is what we do. Lots of little plates to share so you get a taste of everything. This way of eating feels a lot like what the Swedes call *lagom*, translating more or less to "Not too little, not too much. Just right."

In honour of my distant Scandinavian heritage, I dedicate this chapter to exactly that. A little bit of everything. Not too much, not too little. Just right.

In this chapter you'll find all sorts of dishes that stand alone as a lunch or light dinner, plates that go well together to create a tapas-style menu, and even some nibbles and canapés. From the show-stopper Beetroot Salmon Gravadlax with Pickled Cucumber (p 82) to the Chicken, Leek and Ginger Potstickers (p 62), my Munchies 3 Ways (p 88) to the warming Roasted Tomato and Pepper Soup with Kale and Pistachio Pesto (p 58), these are recipes you'll make time and time again.

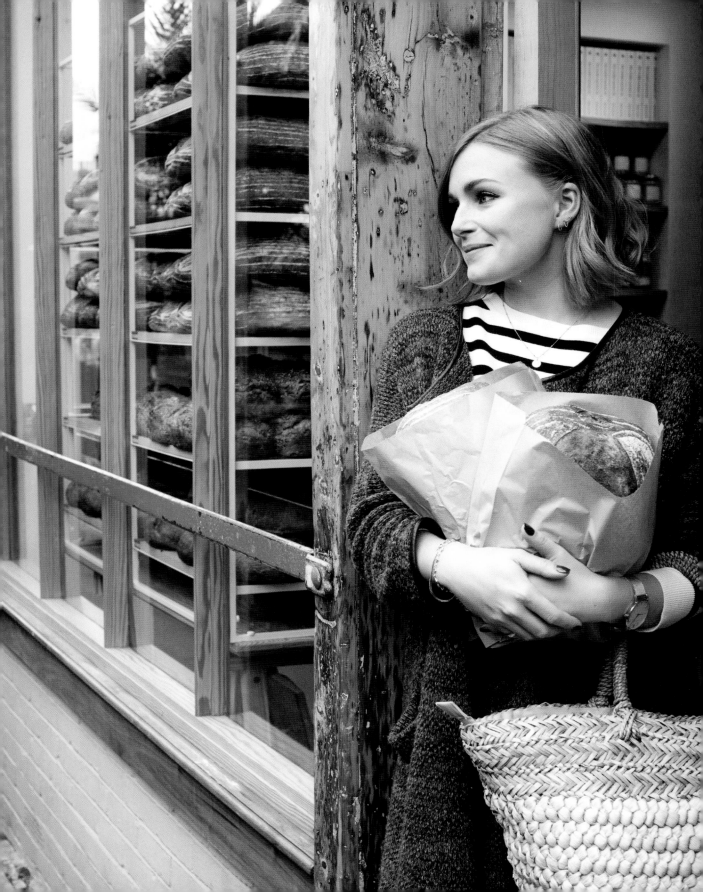

ROASTED TOMATO AND PEPPER SOUP
WITH KALE AND PISTACHIO PESTO

SERVES
4

This is one of my all-time favourite soups for the winter months and it really hits the spot. An oldie but a goodie, and reassuringly hearty when finished off with creamy crème fraîche and a dollop of Kale and Pistachio Pesto (p 191).

INGREDIENTS:

800g red tomatoes,
roughly chopped
2 yellow peppers, deseeded
and roughly chopped
1 red onion, thickly sliced
2 sprigs of fresh thyme
4 tbsp olive oil
500ml hot vegetable stock
2 tbsp crème fraîche
4 tsp Kale and Pistachio Pesto
(see page 191)
extra-virgin olive oil,
for drizzling
sea salt and freshly ground
black pepper

METHOD:

Preheat the oven to 200°C/180°C fan/Gas mark 6.

Throw the tomatoes, peppers, onion and thyme into a baking tray. Drizzle generously with olive oil and season well with salt and pepper. Give it a stir and pop in the oven to cook for 30–35 minutes until soft and browned.

Remove the tray from the oven, discard the thyme stalks, and place the vegetables into a blender along with the stock, and blitz. Check you're happy with the consistency and flavour, adding more seasoning or stock if necessary. Add most of the crème fraîche and blitz once more until combined.

Pour into bowls, swirl a teaspoon each of crème fraîche and kale and pistachio pesto into the soup and finish with a drizzle of extra-virgin olive oil.

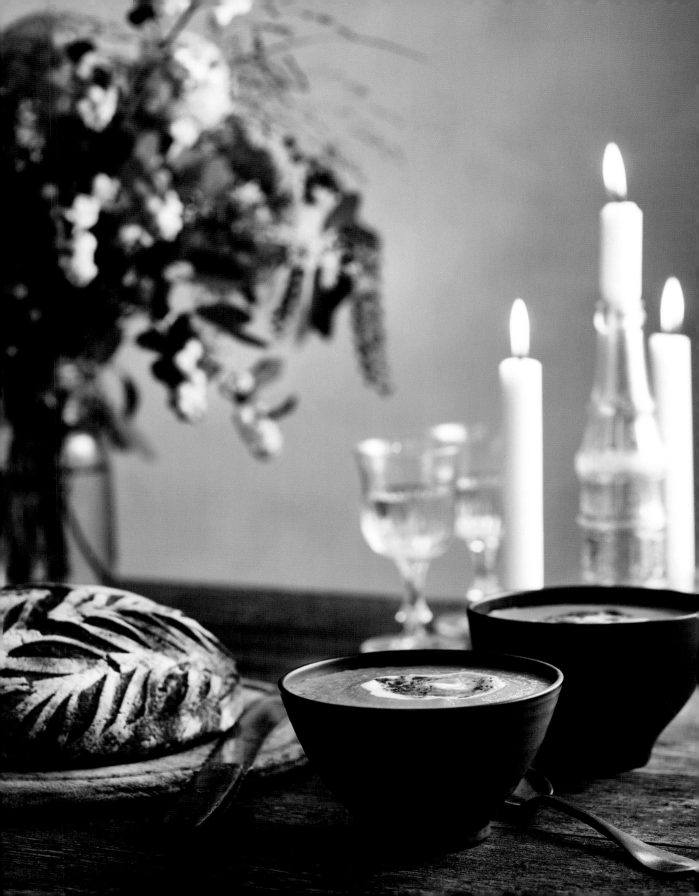

SPICY ASIAN CHICKEN WINGS

SERVES
2 – 4

Chicken wings have always been, and will continue to be, my Number 1 guilty pleasure. These wings have a sticky hot, spicy and sweet sauce that's so moreish you'll be wanting to make another batch straight away. If you have a kitchen thermometer, it would be handy here but isn't essential.

INGREDIENTS:

2 tbsp gochujang Korean chili paste (available online or at Asian supermarkets)

1 tbsp Sriracha chilli sauce (available at all large supermarkets)

4 tbsp soft brown sugar

3 tbsp malt vinegar

2 tbsp tomato ketchup

2 tbsp barbecue sauce

1 tsp American hot sauce

1 tbsp sesame oil

1 tbsp butter

1 tsp salt

4 tbsp plain flour

4 tbsp cornflour

12 chicken wings, patted dry with kitchen towel

vegetable oil, for deep-frying enough to fill a pan up to ⅓

black sesame seeds

spring onion, finely sliced

1 red chilli, finely sliced

METHOD:

To make the sauce, place a pan over a medium–high heat and add the gochujang, Sriracha chilli sauce, sugar, vinegar, ketchup, barbecue sauce, American hot sauce, sesame oil, butter and salt. Bring to the boil and allow to bubble for a couple of minutes, then remove from the heat and set aside.

Mix the plain flour and cornflour in a bowl and season with a big pinch of salt. Toss the wings in the flour mix until fully coated.

Heat the vegetable oil in a heavy-based saucepan to 140°C or until the edge of a chicken wing sizzles in the oil. Carefully add the wings and fry for 8–10 minutes or until they are cooked through but still pale in colour.

Transfer the wings onto kitchen paper and scatter with more flour. Increase the temperature of the oil to 190°C (or simply turn up the heat, if you don't have a thermometer, and wait for 5 minutes), return the wings to the pan and fry for a further 2–3 minutes until golden.

Drain the wings on kitchen paper before coating in the spicy sauce. Scatter over the sesame seeds, red chilli and spring onion and serve immediately.

CLAMS
WITH PANCETTA AND CIDER

SERVES

4

Clams are my favourite shellfish. I eat them by the bucket-load when I go abroad and live off them when I go on holiday to Portugal. These are a different take on the classic lemon, garlic and white wine clams, using something a bit more British: bacon and cider. This dish is sweet, tangy and salty and needs only a spoon and a wedge of bread to mop up all the delicious sauce.

INGREDIENTS:

4 rashers streaky pancetta, sliced

1 tbsp olive oil

1 banana shallot, sliced

1 garlic clove, crushed

150ml dry cider

juice of ½ lemon

500g fresh clams, left to sit in a bowl of cold water for at least 30 minutes

extra-virgin olive oil, for drizzling

1 tbsp flat-leaf parsley, finely chopped

sea salt and freshly ground black pepper

METHOD:

In a heavy-based pan, heat the olive oil over a medium heat and throw in the pancetta. Fry for a few minutes until lightly golden brown and crispy, then remove from the pan and drain on kitchen paper.

Add the shallot to the pan and turn down the heat, cooking for a few minutes until soft. Add the garlic and cook for another couple of minutes.

Pour in the cider and the lemon juice and bring to the boil.

Drain the clams, discarding any that are open or damaged. Add the clams to the pan, reduce to a simmer and cover. Leave to cook for 3–5 minutes, or until all the shells have opened. Discard any clams that have not opened after 5 minutes.

Return the pancetta to the pan, check the seasoning and serve with a drizzle of extra-virgin olive oil and chopped parsley.

CHICKEN, LEEK AND GINGER POTSTICKERS

MAKES
24

INGREDIENTS:

800g chicken mince
1 large leek, thinly sliced
1 tsp fresh ginger,
finely chopped
1 tsp garlic, finely chopped
1 tsp toasted sesame oil
1 medium free-range egg,
separated
24 wanton wrappers
(available online or at Asian
supermarkets)
2 tbsp light soy sauce
2 tbsp rice wine vinegar,
(malt vinegar is fine too)
a thumb-sized piece of ginger,
peeled and sliced into
matchsticks
4 tbsp groundnut or vegetable
oil – 1tbsp per batch of
dumplings
sea salt

These potstickers are essentially dumplings, and have a crispy base while the rest is steam-cooked, giving them a beautifully pillow-soft texture. Make these with a group of friends around the table or make a batch, pop in the freezer, and cook straight from frozen.

METHOD:

In a bowl, mix together the chicken mince, leek, ginger, garlic, sesame oil, egg white and salt.

Lay out the wanton wrappers (not too many at a time, or they'll dry out) and carefully brush the egg yolk around the edge of the wrapper. Spoon a teaspoon of filling into the centre of each wrapper and then bring the curves together to make a half moon shape, without pressing the edges together.

Now create the folds. Press together the edges in the middle of the half moon, then concertina the pastry by pinching along the edge of the pastry on one side of your half moon, beginning from the corner, and working your way into the centre, then joining the edges together. What you will have is a dumpling with pastry that's folded on one side. Make sure there are no gaps and the pastry is fully bonded. Repeat with the remaining dumplings.

Heat a large, non-stick pan over a medium–high heat and add a tablespoon of oil. Once the oil is hot, place the dumplings into the pan six at a time and quickly fry the bottom of the dumplings for 1 minute.

Very carefully, add 50ml boiling water to the pan and cover. (If you have a bamboo lid, this is perfect for the job.) Steam for 8–10 minutes. (If cooking from frozen, allow a further 4–5 minutes steaming.)

Remove the lid and allow the dumplings to cook for a further few minutes in the pan until all of the water has evaporated and the dumplings start frying again to form a crust.

Transfer the dumplings to a serving dish. Combine the soy sauce, vinegar and ginger in a dipping bowl and serve immediately.

These dumplings can be stored in the freezer, in a freezer bag quite happily for 4 months.

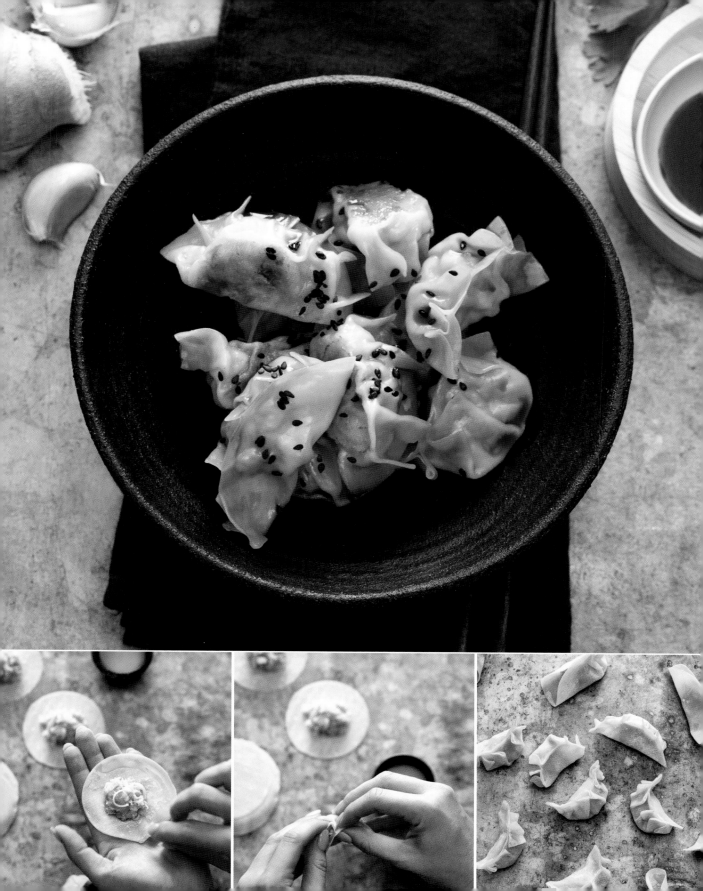

RAINBOW SALAD ROLLS
WITH TANGY PEANUT DIP

These rolls are super-easy to make and look really rather pretty. It's up to you what you put in them. If you like meat, then don't hold back; chuck in some cooked beef and chicken. If you're a fish person, then go for prawns, it all works just as well. These are how I like to eat mine, as a light snack, a starter or as an accompaniment to a main meal.

MAKES
4

INGREDIENTS:

1 carrot
1 cucumber
1 iceberg lettuce
4 rice paper wraps (available at most major supermarkets in the Asian section)
a handful of fresh coriander leaves
1 red pepper, deseeded and thinly sliced
1 yellow pepper, deseeded and thinly sliced
¼ red cabbage, thinly sliced
2 tbsp Tangy Peanut Dip (see page 194)
1 tbsp salted peanuts, crushed

METHOD:

Using a vegetable peeler or a julienne peeler, peel the carrot and cucumber into ribbons or shreds. Carefully peel the iceberg leaves off the lettuce head, leaving them whole and resembling bowls. Keep everything in separate piles to make it easier to assemble.

One at a time, hold the rice paper wraps under the cold tap until pliable and lay down on a chopping board.

Place a few coriander leaves on the rice paper and then lay an iceberg lettuce leaf on top. Lay small bundles of the sliced vegetables horizontally in the middle of the lettuce leaf.

Fold in the right and left side of the wrap by 2–3cm, and then from the bottom up, roll the wrap into a spring roll, securing the end with a little water.

Leave the spring rolls whole, or slice in half and serve with the Tangy Peanut Dip and crushed peanuts.

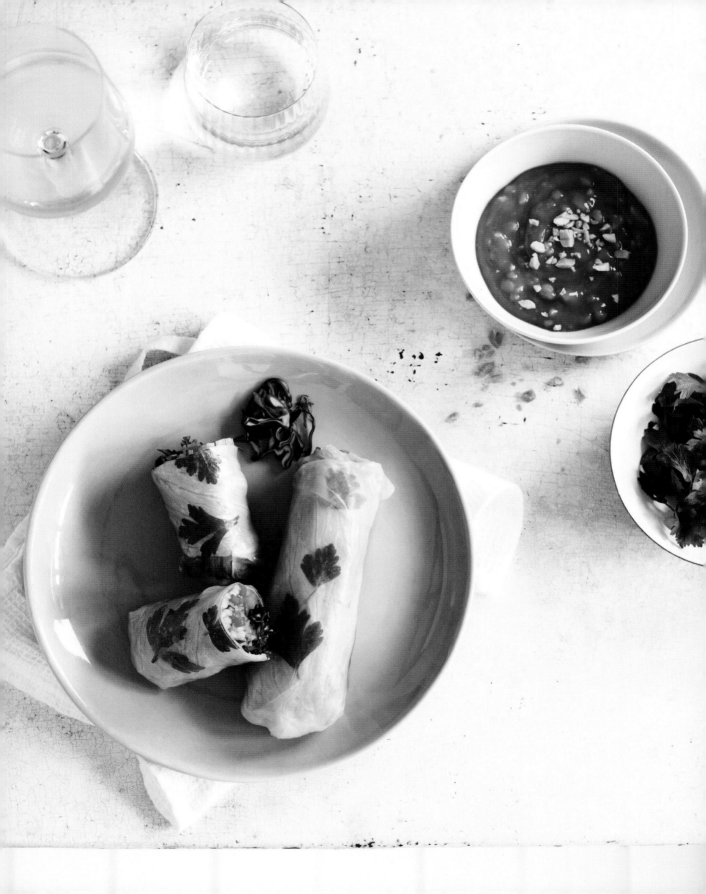

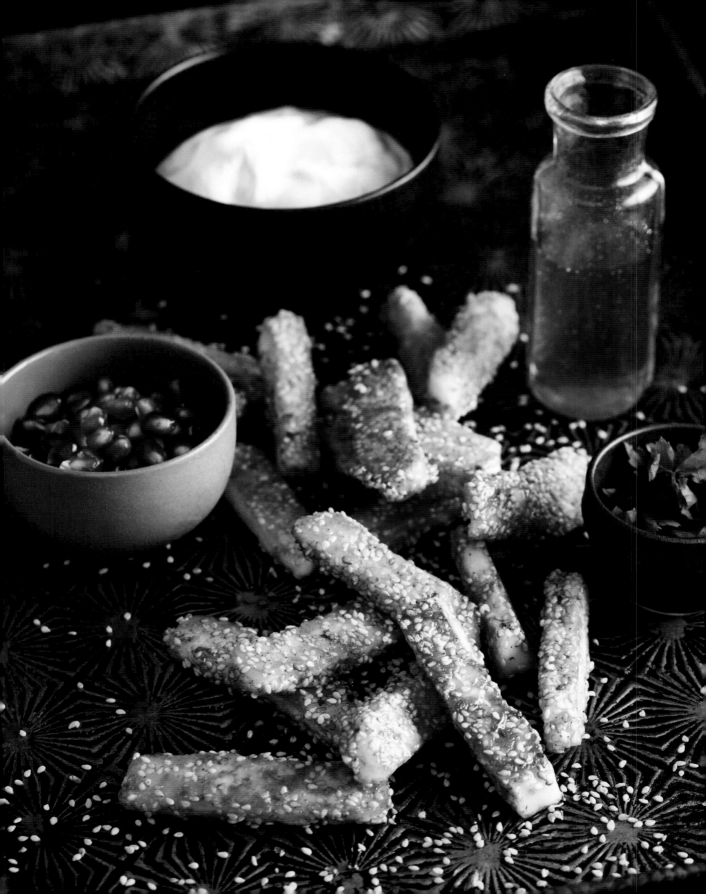

HALLOUMI FRIES
WITH SOURED CREAM, HONEY AND POMEGRANATE

SERVES
2

Since making these, I have never looked back. Halloumi fries coated in a crispy layer of sesame seeds and served with sour cream, honey and fresh pomegranate – you'd be forgiven for thinking you're in the Mediterranean. These are a great starter or light lunch but also work very well alongside other dishes if you're cooking up a feast.

INGREDIENTS:

4 tbsp plain flour
1 tsp sesame seeds
1 x 250g pack of halloumi cut into chunky chip "fries"
vegetable oil, for deep-frying
1 tsp honey
seeds of ½ pomegranate
1 bunch of flat-leaf parsley
4 tbsp soured cream

METHOD:

In a bowl combine the flour and sesame seeds. Coat the halloumi fries in the mixture until covered.

Place a small heavy-based pan over a medium–high heat and pour in 2–3cm of vegetable oil. Test to see if the oil is ready by dropping a small piece of halloumi into the pan. It should immediately start sizzling.

Carefully place a few halloumi fries in the pan and fry for a couple of minutes on each side until crunchy and golden. You'll need to do this in batches of 4 or 5 so as not to overcrowd the pan.

Using a slotted spoon, carefully remove the fries and drain on kitchen paper.

Drizzle the halloumi fries with honey, scatter with pomegranate seeds and parsley and serve with a dollop of soured cream on the side.

PAN-FRIED GNUDI
WITH A CREAMY GORGONZOLA SAUCE

SERVES
4

Gnudi are simply cheese balls! If you're a fan of cheese like me, then this is the ultimate recipe. Ricotta and Parmesan rolled into balls and slathered in a blue cheese sauce. Utter heaven. There's a bit of pre-preparation involved – it will take 24 hours all in – but trust me, the results are worth it. Get the best-quality ricotta that you can afford, or you'll end up with a soggy mess. As long as the ricotta is dry you'll end up with light, fluffy gnudi covered in a rich and creamy sauce.

INGREDIENTS:

250g best quality fresh ricotta
(from an Italian deli if possible)
50g freshly grated Parmesan
nutmeg, freshly grated
a few gratings of lemon zest
250g semolina
50g butter
extra-virgin olive oil, for
drizzling
a few thyme leaves
50g Gorgonzola
sea salt and freshly ground
black pepper

METHOD:

If your ricotta is wet, you will need to strain it. Gently break up the ricotta in a sieve over a bowl and leave in the fridge for at least two hours to drain off any excess moisture. It needs to be dry and crumbly.

Put the ricotta, Parmesan, nutmeg and lemon zest in a bowl and beat together until smooth. Add a pinch of salt and pepper and taste to check the seasoning.

Spread the semolina out on a large baking tray. Grab a small golf-ball sized piece of the ricotta mixture and roll between your hands to form a ball, then pop it on the semolina. Do this with the remaining mixture, then roll the tray back and forth to gently cover the balls in semolina.

Stick the entire tray, uncovered, in the fridge overnight. The semolina will draw out all the moisture from the ricotta and create a fabulous crust.

Bring a large pan of salted water to the boil, gently drop the gnudi into the water and cook for about 2 minutes or until they have all risen to the surface.

Meanwhile, put a pan over a medium heat and add the butter and a drizzle of olive oil.

Once the butter has melted, rip in most of the thyme leaves and crumble in the Gorgonzola.

Add a tablespoon of the gnudi cooking water and swirl the pan to create a creamy sauce.

Serve the gnudi with the Gorgonzola sauce spooned over and finish with a light drizzle of extra-virgin olive oil and a scattering of thyme leaves.

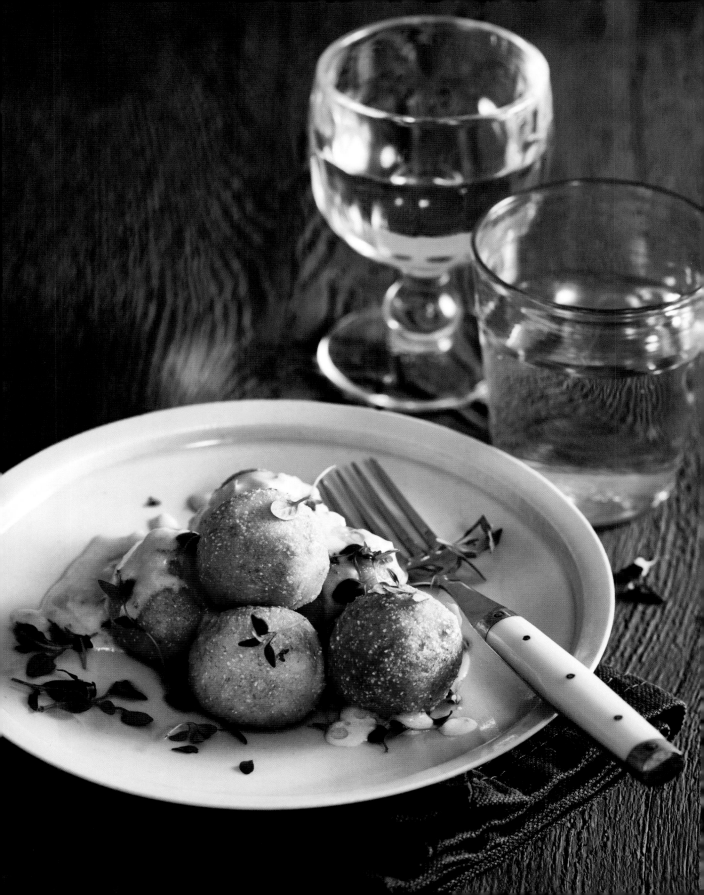

CAULIFLOWER "RICE" SMOKED SALMON SUSHI ROLLS

SERVES
2

Cauliflower rice has been getting a bit of a bad reputation since the clean eating brigade took ownership over it, but I'd like to stress it has been around for a while . . . In fact, before it became a trendy carbohydrate replacement, I was putting it into my mashed potato with garlic and butter to bulk it out! I don't look at this as a "carb-free" version of sushi – I love sushi and eat far too much of it. This is just something a bit different; light, fresher but just as tasty.

INGREDIENTS:

1 head of cauliflower
1 tbsp rice wine vinegar
2 nori sheets
100g smoked salmon,
cut into strips
½ cucumber, cut into strips
soy sauce
sea salt

METHOD:

Separate the florets from the cauliflower and grate or pulse in a food processor until you get a rice-like texture.

Pop in a bowl and cover with clingfilm, and microwave for 4 minutes. Pour the cauliflower rice onto a clean tea towel and allow to cool for a few minutes.

Bring the edges of the tea towel up, wring out any excess water and tip the cauliflower into a bowl. Add the rice wine vinegar and salt, and stir to combine. Allow to cool fully.

To assemble the sushi rolls, lay the nori out horizontally in front of you. Starting at the edge closest to you, spread the cauliflower rice over about a third of the nori. About 2–3cm from the bottom, lay the smoked salmon and cucumber horizontally on top of the rice.

From the bottom, tightly roll up the nori into a tube, sealing the end with a little water.

Slice into 2cm pieces and serve with the soy sauce.

PAPRIKA HUMMUS
WITH BAKED WHOLEWHEAT CRISPS

SERVES
2 – 4 as a snack

There is no need ever to buy hummus – making it is so easy, I promise. From one can of chickpeas you can make triple the quantity that you'd pay much more for in the supermarket. The great thing about hummus is, it's pretty much a blank canvas: you can throw anything in there such as sesame seeds or toasted pinenuts. But this is how I like to eat mine, simple and packed with a smoky punch.

INGREDIENTS:

3 wholewheat wraps

FOR THE HUMMUS:

1 x 210g tin chickpeas, drained
1 garlic clove, roughly chopped
2 tsp smoked paprika, plus
extra for sprinkling
3 tbsp lemon juice
2 tbsp tahini
2 tbsp water
2 tbsp extra-virgin olive oil
sea salt

METHOD:

Preheat the oven to 200°C/180°C fan/Gas mark 6.

Cut each wrap into 8 triangles, place on a baking tray and bake in the oven for 4 minutes on either side.

To make the hummus, combine all the ingredients in a food processor and blend until smooth. Chill in the fridge for at least 1 hour before serving.

Serve with an extra sprinkling of paprika and a drizzle of extra-virgin olive oil.

CHILLED CUCUMBER AND COCONUT SOUP

SERVES
4 as a starter
or 2 as a light bite

This is my other all-time favourite soup, and it really comes into its own in the warmer months. Delicate, refreshing and extremely easy to make, this is perfect served ice-cold.

INGREDIENTS:

100ml Greek yoghurt
125ml vegetable stock
100ml coconut milk
1 cucumber, peeled
juice of ½ lime
sea salt and freshly ground
black pepper

METHOD:

Blend all the ingredients together in a food processor and season to taste.

Pour into bowls and refrigerate for at least 2 hours until chilled.

Garnish with the dill, drizzle with the extra-virgin olive oil and serve.

TO SERVE:

2 tsp finely chopped dill
extra-virgin olive oil,
for drizzling

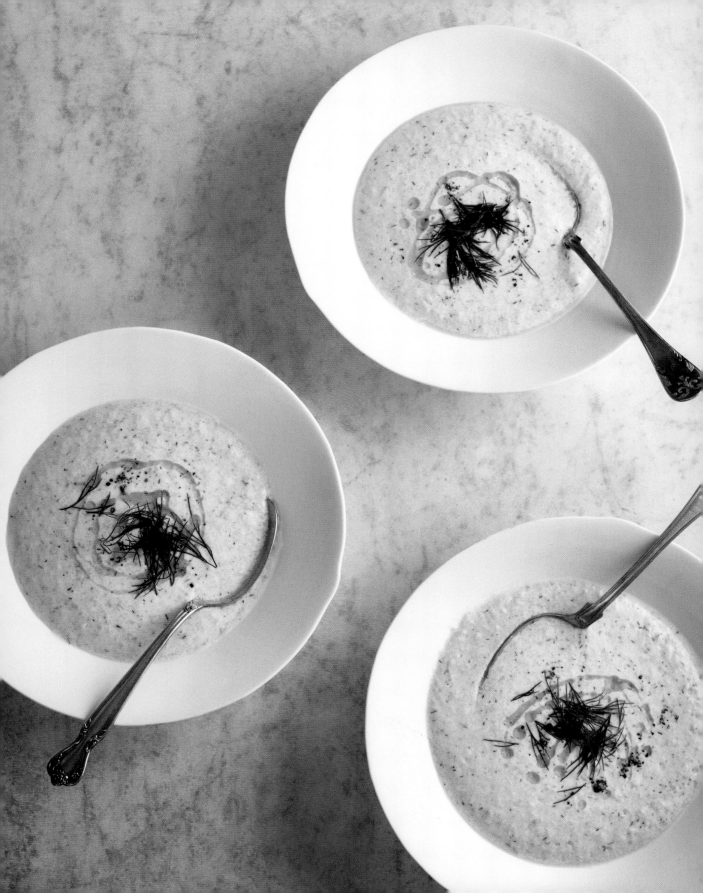

FILO PISSALADIÈRE
WITH SWEET ONIONS, ANCHOVIES AND OLIVES

This is a slightly different take on the classic pissaladière (a traditional French onion tart with anchovies laid along the top in a criss-cross formation) and uses filo pastry instead of a flatbread base. Get a good colour on the onions, and it's plain sailing from then on. It's perfect served with a crisp salad for a light lunch or cut into squares and served as a canapé with drinks.

INGREDIENTS:

1 tbsp olive oil
2 onions, thinly sliced
1 tbsp honey
5 sheets filo pastry
2 tbsp melted butter
1 x 50g tin anchovy fillets
in oil
10 black olives
1 tbsp finely chopped flat-leaf
parsley

METHOD:

Preheat the oven to 200°C/180°C fan/Gas mark 6.

Heat the olive oil in a pan over a medium heat and gently fry the onions for 10 minutes until they are browned and caramelised. Add the honey, stir and set aside to cool.

On a non-stick baking sheet lay down a sheet of filo pastry. Brush with the melted butter and lay down a second, continuing this process until all 5 pastry sheets are sandwiched together.

Brush the edges of the pastry with butter and fold towards the centre to form a border.

Spread the onions out evenly over the base. Place the anchovies over the onions in criss-crosses to create a diamond pattern. Place an olive in the centre of each diamond.

Bake the pissaladière in the oven for 10–12 minutes or until the pastry is golden brown and crisp. Sprinkle over the parsley and serve.

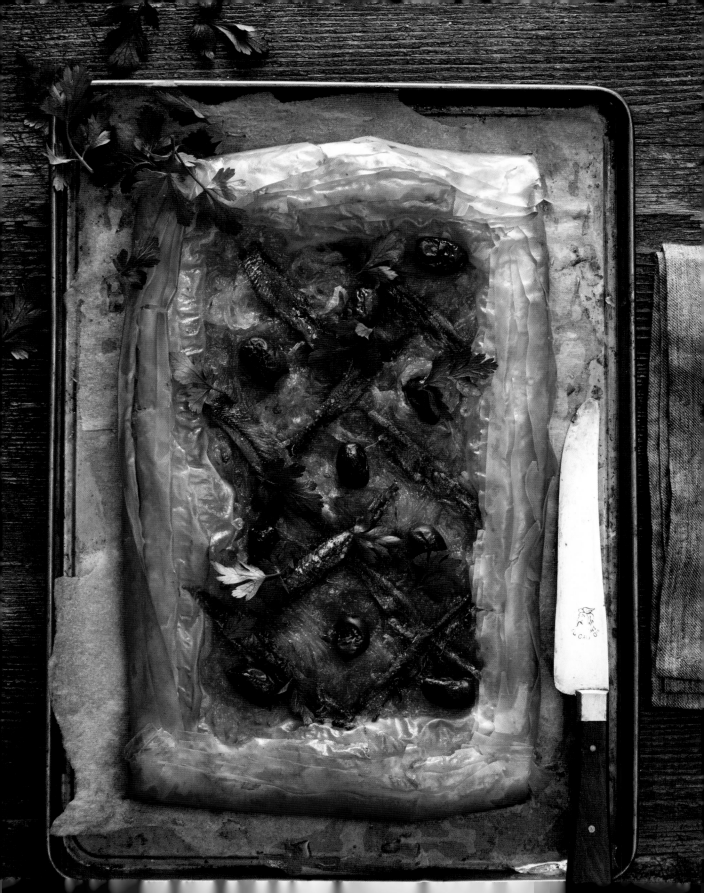

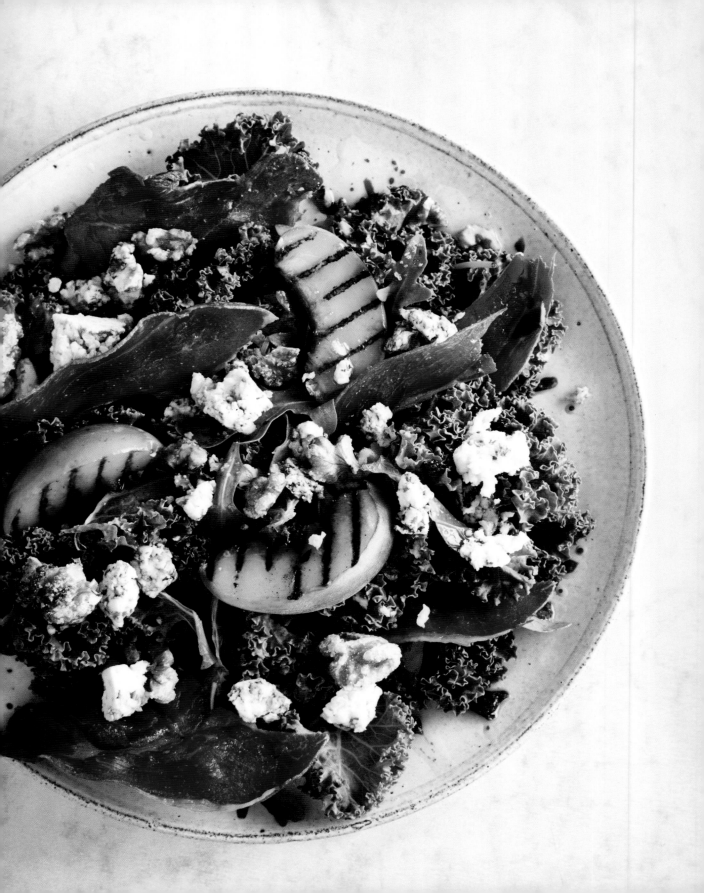

GRILLED PEACH, PROSCIUTTO AND GORGONZOLA SALAD
WITH FROSTED WALNUTS

SERVES
6

When in season, peaches are one of the most delicious fruits, and when they're chargrilled they release a gorgeous caramelised flavour. Teamed with a tangy blue cheese and sweet frosted walnuts, this is the mother of all salads. Perfect as a light lunch or a starter for a dinner party.

INGREDIENTS:

100g walnut halves
25g caster sugar
6 slices prosciutto
olive oil cooking spray
3 large ripe peaches, destoned and sliced into 6 segments
100ml extra-virgin olive oil
50ml balsamic vinegar
1 tbsp honey
200g baby kale or rocket
150g Gorgonzola or any other soft blue cheese
sea salt and pepper

METHOD:

Preheat the oven to 200°C/180°C fan/Gas mark 6. Line a baking sheet with greaseproof paper.

Pop the walnut halves in a bowl with 1 tablespoon water, give them a shake and then drain.

In a clean bowl, toss the walnuts in the caster sugar until fully coated, then scatter over the prepared baking sheet. Bake in the oven for 6–8 minutes until golden brown and frosted. Remove from the oven and allow to cool.

Stick a griddle pan over a medium–high heat, spray the prosciutto with the cooking oil, or lightly brush if you don't have any spray, and cook on the griddle pan for a minute or so on either side until golden brown. Remove from the pan and set aside to cool.

In the same pan, add the sliced peaches and grill for a couple of minutes either side until charred (try not to turn them too often, or you won't get the lovely dark lines on the peaches).

To make the dressing, mix the extra-virgin olive oil, balsamic vinegar, honey, salt and pepper in a bowl, then toss with the baby kale.

Divide the salad between serving plates. Lay an equal number of peach segments on each plate, tear over the prosciutto and arrange the kale on top. Crumble over the Gorgonzola, scatter with the frosted walnuts and serve.

BANG BANG CHICKEN SALAD

SERVES
6

Satay chicken has always been a love of mine and this salad is in homage to that, but teamed with lots of crunchy veg to freshen it up. This recipe lends itself well to being served as a layered salad, or you can go American-style and dice everything up. Either way, serve with lashings of Tangy Peanut Dip and plenty of crispy wonton.

INGREDIENTS:

1 tbsp vegetable oil
6 boneless, skin-on chicken thighs
6 wanton wrappers (or 1 white tortilla wrap if you can't get hold of them)
1 Chinese lettuce (available at all large supermarkets)
½ red cabbage
a large handful of mangetout, sliced into strips
2 spring onions, finely chopped
a handful of fresh coriander leaves, chopped
3 tbsp Tangy Peanut Dip (see page 194)
2 tbsp salted peanuts, crushed
sea salt and freshly ground black pepper

METHOD:

Heat the vegetable oil in a large frying pan over a medium–high heat.

Season the chicken skins with salt and fry the thighs, skin down, for 5–6 minutes until crispy. Turn over and cook for a further 3–4 minutes or until cooked through. Remove the chicken from the pan and slice into strips. Allow to cool.

Shred the wanton wrappers (or tortilla wrap, if using) into 1cm strips, add to the chicken pan and fry for a couple of minutes on each side until crispy. Remove from the pan and drain on kitchen paper.

Shred the Chinese lettuce and red cabbage and put in a large bowl with the mangetout, spring onion, coriander, Tangy Peanut Dip and most of the crushed peanuts. Toss everything together and transfer onto a serving platter.

Top with the sliced chicken and crispy wanton strips and the remaining peanuts, then serve with lime wedges.

TO SERVE:

1 lime, cut into wedges

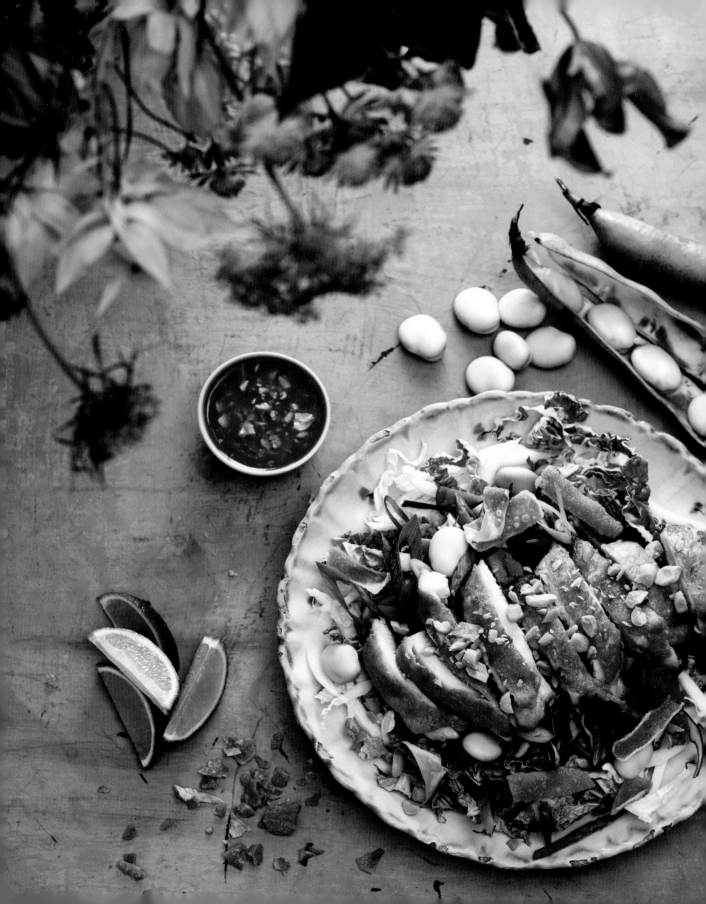

MUSHROOM, RICOTTA AND THYME FILO QUICHE

SERVES
4

I started making quiche with filo pastry and I've never looked back! There's something so incredibly satisfying about super-crisp pastry enveloping a light, fluffy egg filling. The secret to getting a crispy base is using an enamel or metal tin. The heat needs to hit the pastry base fast and evenly, so don't use ceramic, or you'll get a soggy bottom… and nobody likes a soggy bottom.

INGREDIENTS:

2 tbsp butter, melted
6 sheets filo pastry
1 tbsp olive oil
a handful of mushrooms,
chopped (shiitake, chestnut,
whatever you fancy)
3 eggs
250g ricotta cheese
50g Parmesan cheese,
freshly grated
50ml milk
2 sprigs of fresh thyme,
leaves picked
sea salt and freshly ground
black pepper

METHOD:

Preheat the oven to 200°C/180°C fan/Gas mark 6.

Brush a 20cm diameter ovenproof metal tin with the butter and lay one sheet of filo over the top, carefully pressing it into the base of the tin so it fits snugly. Brush the pastry lightly with butter and place another sheet at a slight angle to the first sheet and brush with more butter. Continue this process with all 6 sheets until the filo pastry fans around the tin, leaving the edges draping over the side.

Heat the oil in a pan placed over a high heat and fry the mushrooms until they start to brown. Remove from the heat and allow to cool.

In a bowl, whisk together the eggs, ricotta, Parmesan, milk, salt and pepper, then pour over the filo base. Scatter over the mushrooms and thyme leaves and bake in the oven for 25–30 minutes.

Once cooked, remove from the oven and allow to set for at least 10 minutes before removing from the tin.

STICKY CALAMARI
WITH GINGER AND CORIANDER

SERVES
2

This is such a cracking dish. Comforting, tasty, sticky and surprisingly easy to make. Do try to get hold of some fresh squid, either from your local fishmonger or supermarket. Ask them to gut them for you, and you won't be faced with black squid ink all over your kitchen (I've been there). But if not, frozen is fine.

INGREDIENTS:

2 whole squid, gutted
and cleaned
100g cornflour
2 egg whites, beaten
a handful of fresh coriander
leaves, chopped, plus a few left
whole for garnish
a 2.5cm piece of ginger cut
into pieces
1 heaped tbsp oyster sauce
2 tsp caster sugar
1 tsp ground black pepper
vegetable or sunflower oil,
for deep-frying
sea salt and freshly ground
black pepper

METHOD:

Using a sharp knife, cut along one side of the squid. Open it out flat on the chopping surface, laying the inner tube downwards. Lightly score the top in diagonal lines. Cut into 4cm x 2cm strips.

Place the cornflour in a bowl and add the salt and pepper. Dip the squid strips in the egg white and then coat in flour mixture, shaking off any excess.

Heat the vegetable or sunflower oil in a heavy-based pan placed over a high heat – the oil is hot enough when a little bit of batter dropped into the oil sizzles straight away. Fry the squid strips for a minute on each side, then remove from the pan using a slotted spoon and drain on kitchen paper.

Place the coriander, ginger, oyster sauce, sugar and pepper in a blender with 2 tablespoons water and blitz to form a paste.

Transfer the paste to a pan placed over a medium heat and simmer for a few minutes until sticky. Remove from the heat and toss the squid pieces in the sticky sauce.

Serve immediately with the coriander leaves sprinkled on top.

BEETROOT SALMON GRAVADLAX
WITH PICKLED CUCUMBER

SERVES
12

The Scandinavian in me couldn't resist this dish, which has the most beautiful ombre effect from the beetroot. It's perfect for a get-together or dinner party and makes an elegant starter. A little work and preparation is needed, but that's completely worth it for the wow factor alone.

INGREDIENTS:

1.2kg (or thereabouts) side of fresh salmon, skin on, de-boned

FOR THE FIRST MARINADE:

4 beetroots, peeled and quartered
zest of 3 unwaxed lemons
3 tbsp caster sugar
8 tbsp flaked sea salt
100ml vodka

FOR THE SECOND MARINADE:

8 tbsp dill, roughly chopped
100ml vodka
4 tbsp grated horseradish from a jar

FOR THE PICKLED CUCUMBER:

1 cucumber
1 tsp sea salt
50g caster sugar
60ml white wine vinegar
1 tbsp dill, roughly chopped

METHOD:

In a food processor, blitz the beetroot and lemon zest until they form a paste. Tip into a bowl and mix in the caster sugar, sea salt and vodka.

Lay the salmon in a large baking tray skin-side down and spoon the marinade over the top, making sure you have an even layer covering the salmon. Cover the tray with clingfilm and pop in the fridge overnight.

The following day, transfer the salmon to a board and wipe off any excess marinade. Rinse the baking tray and then pop the salmon back in skin-side down.

Combine the second marinade ingredients in a bowl and spread evenly over the salmon. Cover with clingfilm again, and place back in the fridge for another 12 hours.

To make the pickled cucumber, shave the cucumber into ribbons using a vegetable peeler. Transfer to a bowl and sprinkle with salt and set aside for 10 minutes.

When the time is up, rinse the cucumber ribbons well with cold water, then drain. Return them to the bowl, add the sugar, white wine vinegar and dill and mix well. Transfer to a glass jar and refrigerate before serving. They will keep for up to a week in the fridge.

To serve, use a sharp knife to thinly slice the salmon and serve with the pickled cucumber ribbons.

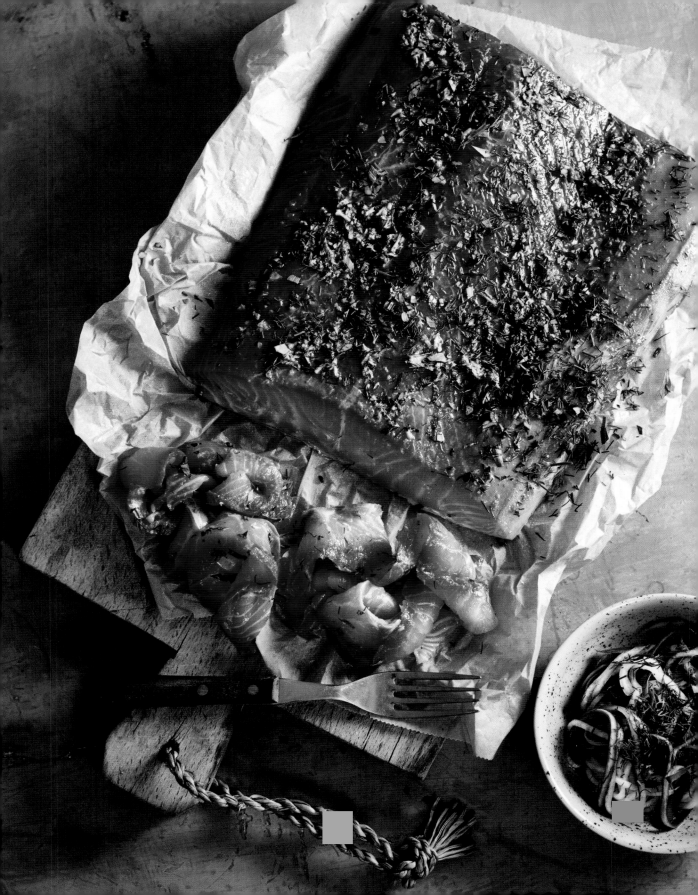

CHARGRILLED PRAWNS WITH LEMON AND CHILLI

SERVES

2

Quick and healthy dinners have never been so in demand! Which is why this dish is a favourite in my house. There's no need to get expensive fresh prawns; many supermarkets sell large packs of king prawns in the freezer section. Take as many out as you need and pop the rest back in the freezer for later.

INGREDIENTS:

225g raw shell-on king prawns

1 tsp olive oil

1 lime, halved

20g flaked sea salt

1 tsp chilli powder

1 tsp lemon zest

a pinch of black pepper

METHOD:

Place a griddle pan over a medium–high heat. Put the prawns in a bowl and toss in the olive oil.

Once the griddle pan is hot, throw in the prawns and cook for a 3–4 minutes on one side, without moving them, and then turn over and cook for another 3–4 minutes. Once nicely pink and charred, remove the prawns from the pan and transfer to a serving dish. Add the lime halves to the pan, cut-side down, pressing them down to achieve char marks.

In a small bowl, combine the salt, chilli powder, lemon zest and pepper and serve alongside the prawns.

STILTON, PEAR AND CARAMELISED ONION TARTS

SERVES
2

Stilton and pear has to be one of my favourite flavour combinations. The perfect easy starter or make-ahead dinner with a crisp green salad.

INGREDIENTS:

1 x 375g pack ready-rolled shortcrust pastry
2 tbsp caramelised onion chutney from a jar
2 eggs – 1 beaten, 1 left whole
2 tbsp crème fraîche
100g Stilton cheese
1 pear, cored and cut into matchsticks

METHOD:

Preheat the oven to 200°C/180°C fan/Gas mark 6.

Line a baking tray with greaseproof paper. Roll out the pastry sheet, cut in half, and lay both halves on the tray. Fold the edges of each half in by 1cm to create a border, and prick the centre of each a few times with a fork. Spread the base of both tarts with the onion chutney.

Crack the whole egg into a bowl, add the crème fraîche and mix well. Carefully spoon the mixture over the bases of the tarts. Crumble over the Stilton and brush the sides of the tart with the beaten egg.

Bake in the oven for 20–25 minutes or until the middle is set and the pastry is golden brown.

Remove from the oven and allow to cool fully before scattering the tarts with the pear matchsticks.

PORK, CRANBERRY AND SAGE SAUSAGE ROLLS

MAKES
12

Why buy sausage rolls when you can make them really easily and pimp them to make them extra tasty? I created these using Mike's leftover Christmas stuffing one year, but they're delicious all year round. They're best straight out of the oven with a side order of my Quick Tomato Chutney (p 50). Also a great packed lunch the next day… if they last that long.

INGREDIENTS:

400g good-quality
sausage meat
30g dried cranberries
zest of 1 orange
a few sage leaves, finely
chopped
1 x 375g pack ready-rolled
puff pastry
plain flour for dusting
1 egg, beaten

METHOD:

Preheat the oven to 200°C/180°C fan/Gas mark 6.

In a bowl, combine the sausage meat, cranberries, orange zest and sage leaves and set aside.

Flour your work surface and lay out the puff pastry sheet in front of you, portrait way up, and cut it in half top to bottom. Halve the sausage mixture and form two long sausages down the middle of each piece of pastry.

Starting with the first half, roll the left-hand side of the pastry over the sausage meat to create a tube and repeat the process with the other half of pastry.

Place the rolls seam side down and using a very sharp knife, carefully cut each of the rolls into six pieces. Lightly score the top of each sausage roll, brush with the beaten egg and transfer onto greaseproof paper on a baking tray. Pop in the oven and bake for 20–25 minutes until golden brown.

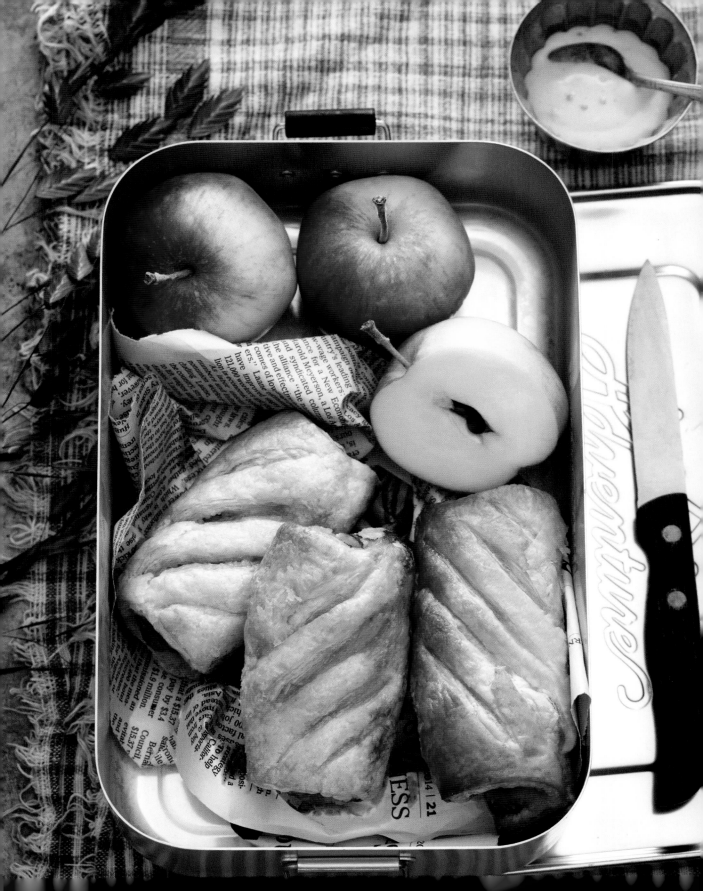

MILLY'S MUNCHIES 3 WAYS:

MAKES
12

When the idea of the same old smoked salmon canapés feels dull and uninspired, why not try something a little different? My munchies are perfect for picnics, party canapés or snacks. All can be pre-made, then cooked as you need them. Try the salmon bites for something a little more refined or the sausage bites with a beer watching TV, and make the arancini with leftover risotto.

PANKO SALMON AND CREAM CHEESE BITES
WITH DILL AND MUSTARD MAYO

INGREDIENTS:

200g cooked salmon flakes (hot smoked, if you can get it)
150g cream cheese
zest of ½ unwaxed lemon
2 tbsp plain flour
1 egg, beaten
4 tbsp finely crushed corn tortilla chips
500ml vegetable oil, for deep-frying
3 tbsp mayonnaise
1 tsp finely chopped dill
1 tsp wholegrain mustard
sea salt and freshly ground black pepper

METHOD:

In a bowl, mix together the salmon, cream cheese, lemon zest, salt and pepper. The mixture will be quite wet, but that's fine.

Divide the mixture into 12 balls. Roll each ball in the flour, then the egg, and then the tortilla crumbs, ensuring they're fully coated. Pop onto a baking tray lined with greaseproof paper and chill in the fridge for at least an hour.

To fry, heat the oil in a deep-fat fryer or heavy-based pan placed over a high heat. Drop a tortilla crumb into the oil to see if it's hot enough; it should sizzle.

Cook the bites in batches of three and transfer onto kitchen paper. Allow to cool for a few minutes.

Meanwhile make the dill and mustard mayo by combining the mayonnaise, dill, mustard, salt and pepper.

Serve immediately.

continued overleaf

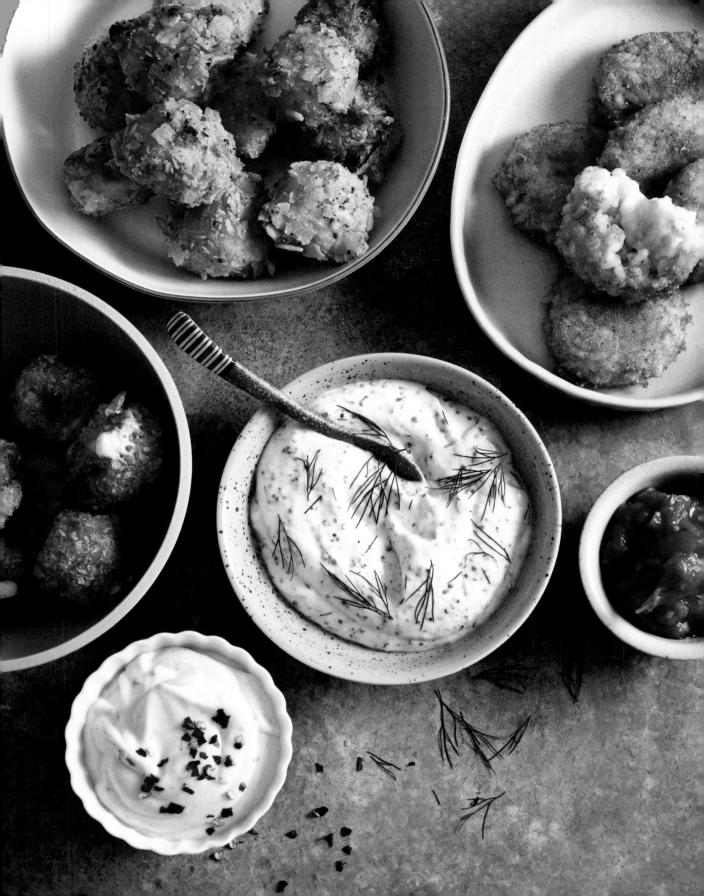

MAKES
12

MOLTEN SAUSAGE BALLS WITH HOT SAUCE MAYO

INGREDIENTS:

2 tbsp mayonnaise

a few drops of hot sauce

400g good-quality sausage meat

100g mature Cheddar, cut into 12 cubes

2 tbsp plain flour

1 egg, beaten

4 tbsp panko breadcrumbs

500ml vegetable oil, for deep-frying

sea salt and freshly ground black pepper

METHOD:

To make the hot sauce mayo, season the mayonnaise with salt and pepper and add a few drops of hot sauce to taste.

Divide the sausage meat into 12 and roll into balls.

Take a piece of sausage meat and make a flat patty in the palm of your hand. Pop a cube of Cheddar in the middle and fold the sausage meat around it, creating a bite-sized ball.

Roll the sausage ball in the flour, and then the egg, and then the panko breadcrumbs, ensuring it is fully coated. Repeat with the remaining sausage balls.

Heat the oil in a deep-fat fryer or a heavy-based pan placed over a medium–high heat. To check the oil is hot enough, drop some breadcrumbs into the oil; if they sizzle straightaway, it's ready.

Fry the sausage bites in batches and transfer onto kitchen paper.

Serve immediately with the hot sauce mayo for dipping.

MAKES
10

MOZZARELLA STUFFED ARANCINI WITH TOMATO SAUCE

INGREDIENTS:

olive oil

1 onion, finely chopped

250g risotto rice

100ml dry Italian white wine

1 litre hot vegetable stock

50g Parmesan cheese,
freshly grated

1 tsp lemon juice

1 ball of fresh mozzarella, torn into
chunks

3 tbsp plain flour

2 eggs, beaten

6 tbsp panko breadcrumbs

500ml vegetable oil for deep-frying

FOR THE SAUCE:

olive oil

2 garlic cloves, finely sliced

a pinch of chilli flakes

1 x 400g tin cherry tomatoes

a handful of fresh basil leaves,
chopped

1 tsp honey

sea salt and freshly ground
black pepper

METHOD:

If using leftover risotto, go straight to grabbing your chunk of risotto to make a patty.

If not, place a pan over a medium heat and fry the onion in a little olive oil until translucent. Add the rice, stir to fully coat the grains with oil and then pour in the wine. Allow the wine to fully cook away and then ladle by ladle add the vegetable stock until the rice is nearly cooked. Add the Parmesan cheese and lemon juice, cover, and rest for 5 minutes, then spread out over a baking tray and allow to cool fully.

To make the arancini, grab a chunk of risotto and make a flat patty in the palm of your hand. Pop a chunk of mozzarella in the middle and form the rice around the cheese, creating a bite-sized ball. Roll in the flour, then liberally brush it with the beaten egg, fully coating it before dropping it into the breadcrumbs. Roll the ball around and ensure it is fully coated with breadcrumbs.

To fry, heat the oil in a deep-fat fryer/heavy-based pan. Drop some breadcrumbs into the oil to see if it's hot enough; they should sizzle straightaway. Cook the arancini in batches of three or four and transfer onto kitchen paper once done to drain.

To make the quick tomato sauce, heat olive oil in a pan over a medium heat. Add to the oil the garlic and chilli flakes and then the tin of tomatoes. Allow the sauce to bubble away for a few minutes until thickened, then tear in a handful of fresh basil and add 1 teaspoon honey and a good pinch of salt and pepper. Serve with the arancini immediately.

There is something so lovely about having friends around: all the candles lit; music playing in the background; shoes off and everyone kicking back on the sofa with a good bottle of wine. Although I like to host and cook for friends, sometimes life gets in the way and I just don't have the time to make a full three-course meal. On these days I make just a few nibbles so we can all have something to eat with our drinks, but I don't have to slave away in the kitchen beforehand. Make as much or as little as you fancy, but these are my go-tos. To make it an absolute doddle, get ahead by preparing the hummus, salmon and cream cheese bites (ready to be fried), truffles and cupcakes in the morning.

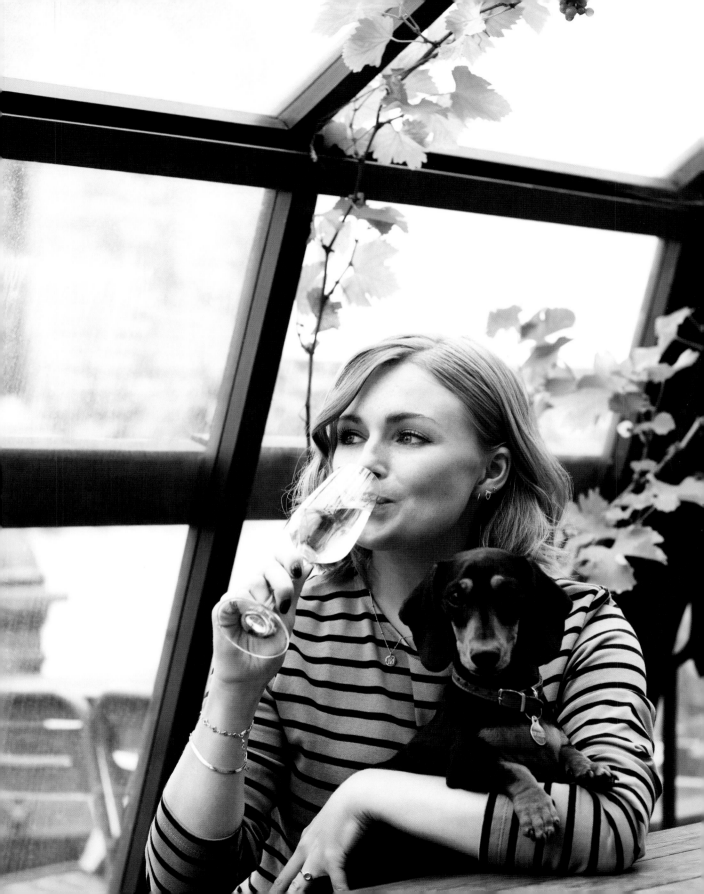

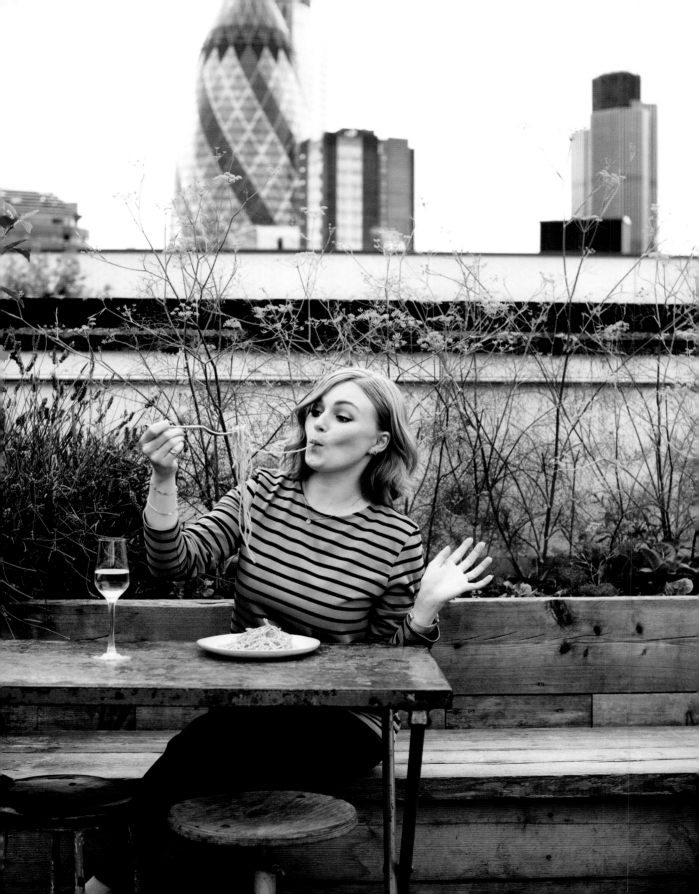

MAINS

"I cook with wine. Sometimes I even add it to the food."
W.C. Fields

For this chapter I've taken inspiration from all the seasons – the crispness of spring, the laziness of summer and the cozy blanket of winter – as well as from across the globe – Asia to the Mediterranean, Scandinavia to Great Britain – and I hope some recipes here whet your appetite.

Above all, the recipes in this chapter fill me with that warm fuzzy autumnal feeling. From a Slow-cooked Oxtail Ragu with Parmesan Mash and Gremolata Oil (p 129), to Sweet and Sticky Pork Ribs (p 124), this chapter is all about "a little bit of what you fancy".

I'm a big fan of arranging impromptu dinner parties, so naturally, I've catered for this too. Moroccan Shepherd's Pie (p 127), Harissa Lamb Meatballs with Bulgur Wheat, Mint and Yoghurt (p 104), One-Pot Sticky Sausage and Three-Bean Cassoulet (p 131) and a special appearance in the form of Mike's Paella (p 112) can all be bulked-up easily to cater for the masses at lunch or supper.

For something lighter during the hotter months, Pan-fried Sea Bass Fillets with Burnt Butter and Caper Sauce (p 103), Asian Beef Lettuce Cups (p 118) and Creamy Saffron and Prosecco Mussels (p 134) are all mouth-wateringly good and not at all heavy.

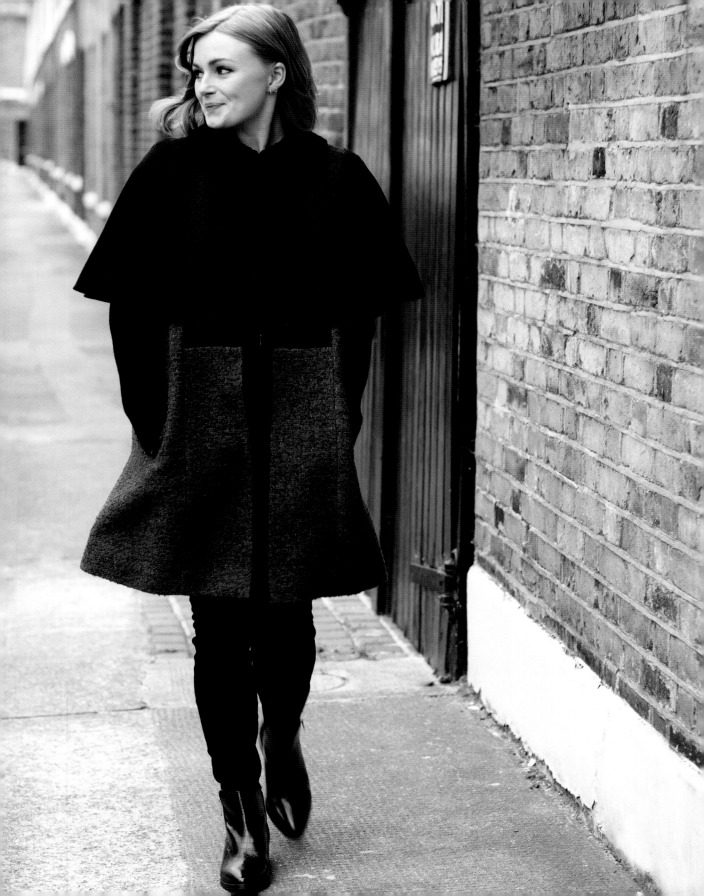

FLOURLESS PIZZA
— HOWEVER YOU LIKE IT

SERVES
1

Cauliflower pizza? I know what you're thinking: a) yuck or b) that's a #CleanEating dish and I don't follow that. Wrong. This pizza has loads of cheese and indulges the dinnertime pizza craving, but without the stodge. Who knew that cauliflower would be the solution to that?

INGREDIENTS:

1 small cauliflower
1 egg
1 tbsp freshly grated
Parmesan cheese
2 tbsp freshly grated hard
mozzarella, plus more for
sprinkling
1 tsp dried oregano, plus more
for sprinkling
1 tsp dried thyme
1 garlic clove, crushed
olive oil
2 tbsp tomato purée loosened
with some water
sea salt and freshly ground
black pepper
any toppings of your choice –
I like fresh mozzarella, my Kale
and Pistachio Pesto (page 191),
prosciutto and freshly grated
Parmesan

METHOD:

Preheat the oven to 220°C/200°C fan/Gas mark 7 and pop in a large baking tray to get piping hot.

Remove the florets from the cauliflower and grate or pulse in a food processor until you get a couscous consistency.

Pop the cauliflower into a bowl, cover with clingfilm and cook in the microwave on high for 4 minutes. Once done, pour the cauliflower onto a clean tea towel and leave to cool for a few minutes.

Gather up the tea towel and wring out the excess water until you are left with a dry mixture. Tip into a bowl. Add the egg, Parmesan, mozzarella, oregano, thyme and garlic and give everything a good mix.

Lay a piece of baking parchment down and rub in some olive oil to stop the pizza base from sticking. Make a ball with the mixture, then pat it down into a circular pizza shape approximately 3mm thick.

Remove the hot baking tray from the oven, then carefully place the pizza base and baking parchment onto the tray. Cook the base in the oven for 10–12 minutes until lightly golden brown.

Remove the base from the oven, gently spread on the tomato purée and sprinkle over the mozzarella. Add a sprinkle of oregano, salt and pepper and any other toppings you'd like, then pop in the oven for another 5 minutes until the cheeses have melted.

Leave to stand for a few minutes, then cut up and dig in.

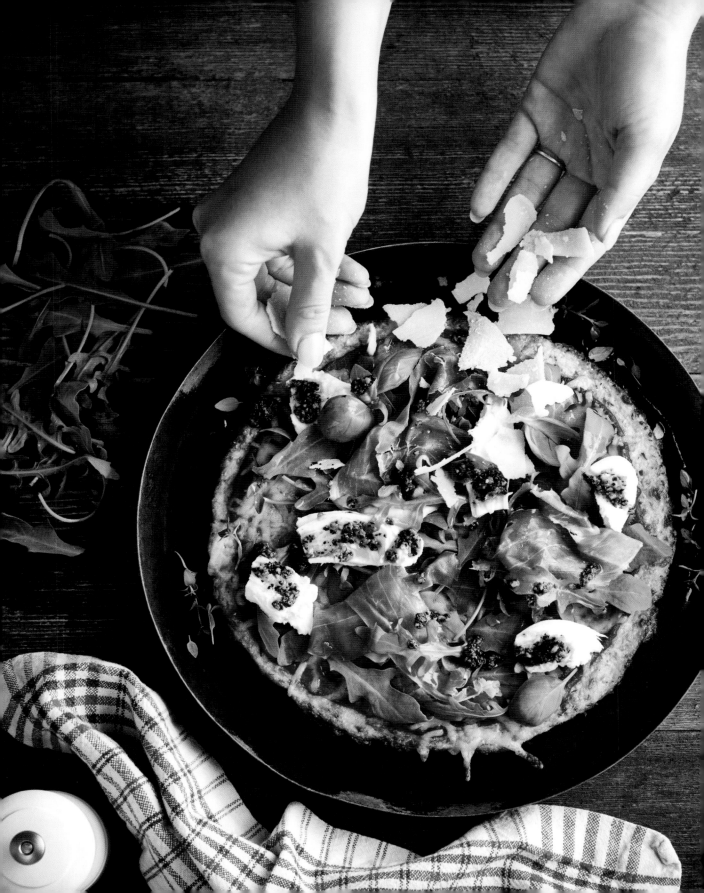

SWEET POTATO GNOCCHI
WITH GARLIC, CHILLI AND ROCKET

Few things are more comforting than a big bowl of gnocchi and it's surprisingly easy to make. I've been making gnocchi from sweet potatoes for years – their sweetness combined with salty butter and Parmesan is divine. This recipe serves 2, but you can easily double or triple the quantities. Once made, the gnocchi will happily sit in the freezer for up to 1 month until you need them.

SERVES
2

INGREDIENTS:

2 sweet potatoes, about 1kg
1 egg
200g plain flour, plus extra
for dusting
olive oil
1 tbsp butter
2 garlic cloves, crushed
½ tsp dried chilli flakes
a handful of rocket leaves
freshly grated Parmesan cheese
– as much as you fancy
sea salt and freshly ground
black pepper

METHOD:

Prick the sweet potatoes with a fork, wrap in damp kitchen paper and microwave separately on high for 8–10 minutes until soft. Carefully cut them in half and allow to cool.

Once cool enough to handle, spoon out the flesh of the sweet potatoes into a large bowl and mash thoroughly with a fork. Add the egg, flour, salt and pepper and combine until it forms a dough that's solid enough to knead. (Some sweet potatoes have a higher moisture content, so you may need to add more flour.)

Flour a work surface and knead the sweet potato dough for a few minutes until you have a smooth dough – this takes up to 10 minutes.

Halve the dough, and roll each half into a long, thin sausage, about the thickness of your thumb. Using a sharp knife, cut into 2.5cm pillows.

Bring a pan of salted water to the boil and cook the gnocchi in two batches for 1 minute.

Using a slotted spoon, remove the gnocchi from pan and drain onto kitchen paper.

Place a non-stick frying pan over a medium–high heat and add a glug of olive oil. Add the gnocchi and cook for a couple of minutes until golden brown on one side. Flip them over and cook the other side for another minute or two until golden brown, then remove from the pan.

Add the butter, garlic and chilli flakes to the pan and fry for a couple of minutes until the garlic has started to brown. Pop the cooked gnocchi back into the pan and add the rocket, then give it all a good stir.

Transfer the gnocchi to bowls and sprinkle with grated Parmesan.

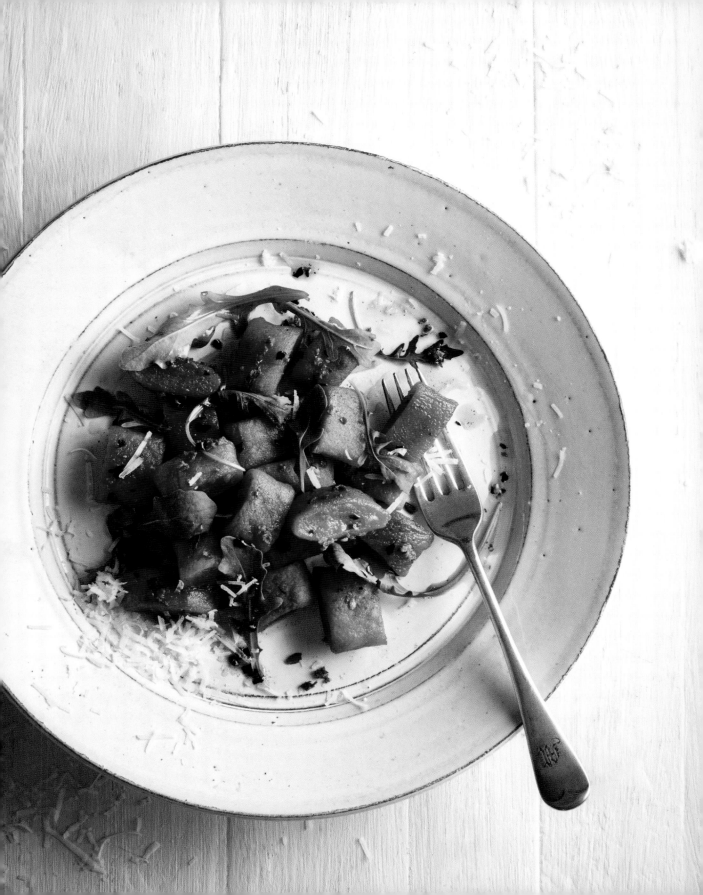

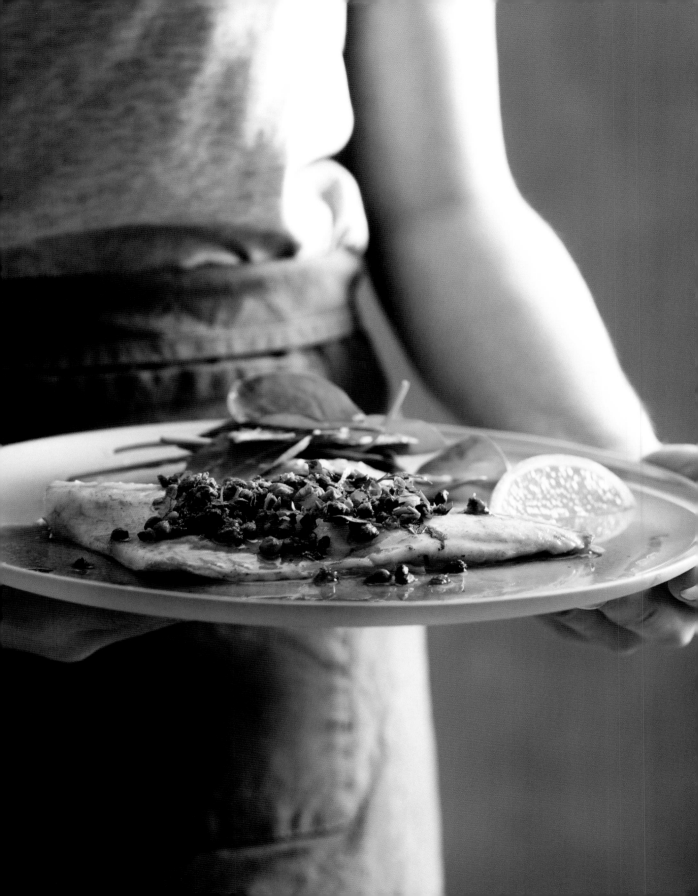

PAN-FRIED SEA BASS FILLETS
WITH BURNT BUTTER AND CAPER SAUCE

SERVES
4

For an amazingly quick and easy but delicious fish recipe that packs a punch, look no further. From pan to plate in less than ten minutes, this is my go-to for a quick and easy supper.

INGREDIENTS:

olive oil
4 boneless seabass fillets
80g salted butter, cubed
2 tbsp small capers, drained
and roughly chopped
zest of ½ unwaxed lemon
1 tsp finely chopped flat-leaf
parsley

METHOD:

Preheat the oven to 110°C/90°C fan/Gas mark ¼.

Heat a glug of olive oil in a large frying pan placed over a high heat. Season the seabass fillets with salt on both sides.

Add two of the fillets to the pan, skin-side down, and cook for about 3 minutes (if you cook them all at once, you will overcrowd the pan and end up with soggy skin). Turn them over and cook for a further 2 minutes. Transfer to the oven to keep warm and repeat with the remaining two fillets. Once all the fillets are cooked, transfer to serving plates and keep warm.

Add the butter to the pan and swirl it around to pick up all of the fish juices. Add the capers and lemon zest and leave the butter to foam and bubble. Once the butter is a nutty brown, spoon over the cooked seabass and scatter with parsley. Serve immediately.

This goes really well with a mixed green salad.

HARISSA LAMB MEATBALLS
WITH BULGUR WHEAT, MINT AND YOGHURT

SERVES
3 – 4

For something a little different, try making your meatballs with lamb and serve them with bulgur wheat instead of rice. Bulgur wheat has a satisfying texture, a bit like chopped up brown rice, and works wonderfully with this dish. The harissa yoghurt is quite mild, so if you like a little more heat, feel free to increase the harissa quantity.

INGREDIENTS:

200g bulgur wheat
500g lamb mince
1 onion, finely chopped
2 garlic cloves, crushed
1 tsp cumin
1 tsp cinnamon
2 tsp harissa paste
2 carrots, finely grated
2 spring onions, finely chopped
1 egg
1 tsp salt
olive oil
juice of ½ lemon
4 tbsp natural yoghurt
a handful of fresh mint,
roughly chopped
extra-virgin olive oil, for
drizzling
1 lemon, cut into wedges

METHOD:

Fill a pan with water and bring to the boil. Add the bulgur wheat and cook for 15 minutes.

In a large bowl combine the lamb, onion, garlic, spices, 1 teaspoon harissa paste, carrot, spring onion, egg and salt. Use your hands to mix everything together really well until combined.

Roll the lamb mixture into balls approximately the size of a twopence-piece – you should get between 15–20 balls in total.

Heat a glug of olive oil in a pan over a medium–high heat and cook the meatballs in batches until browned all over.

Drain the bulgur wheat, add the lemon juice and stir well. Put the yoghurt in a small serving bowl and swirl in the remaining harissa paste.

Scatter the meatballs with the mint and serve with the bulgur wheat and yoghurt. Finish with a drizzle of extra-virgin olive oil and some lemon wedges on the side.

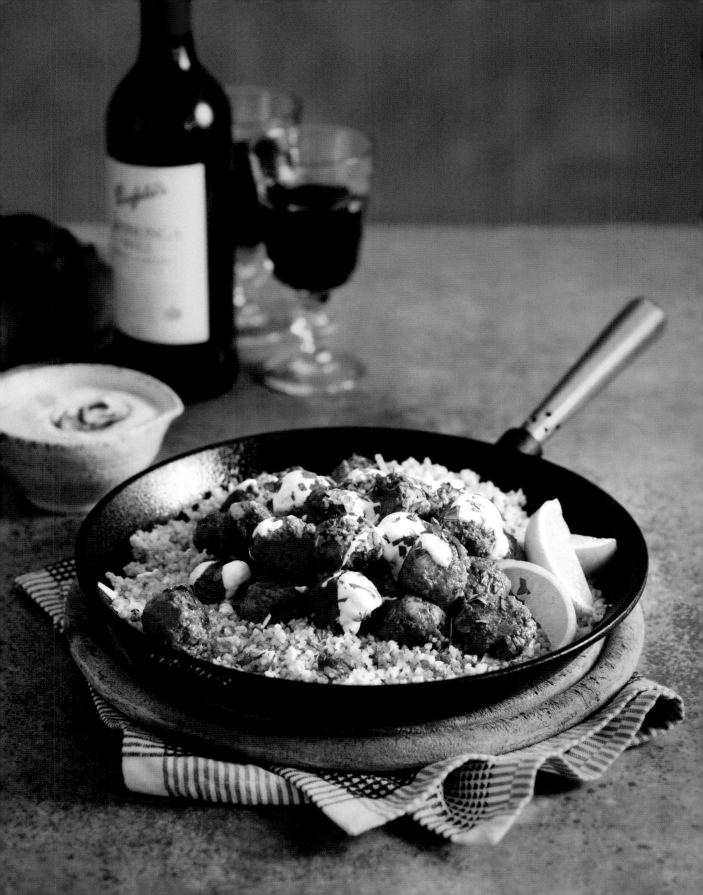

ROAST CHICKEN, LEEK AND BARLEY RISOTTO
WITH THE BEST GRAVY

Sometimes a Sunday roast is too much to cook. I know, I said it! But we've all had those weekends where there's too much to do, and the idea of spending your few hours off in the kitchen is enough to make you pick up a takeaway menu. This dish is the solution – roast chicken and the best gravy fools you into thinking you're having a Sunday roast, but we're serving it with a low maintenance pearl barley risotto. The oven and stove do all the work, and you're not juggling ten pans at once. Result.

INGREDIENTS:

FOR THE CHICKEN AND GRAVY:

1 onion, quartered

2 carrots, roughly chopped

2 celery sticks, roughly chopped

2 garlic cloves, crushed

1 small potato, quartered

olive oil

1 x 1.5kg free-range chicken

½ lemon

a sprig of rosemary

1 tbsp plain flour

100ml red wine

200ml good-quality chicken stock

1 tbsp honey

sea salt and freshly ground black pepper

METHOD:

Preheat the oven to 200°C/180°C fan/Gas mark 6.

Place the onion, carrot, celery, garlic and potato in a large high-top baking tray, and drizzle over some olive oil. Rub the chicken all over with some more olive oil, cover generously with sea salt, then place on top of the vegetables. Pop the lemon and rosemary up the cavity and place on the middle shelf of the oven and cook for approximately 1 hour 20 minutes. (Check the cooking guidelines on the chicken packet, as this will vary depending on its size.)

Around 40 minutes into the chicken cooking time, start the pearl barley risotto. Heat 1 tablespoon olive oil in a large, heavy-based pan placed over a medium heat. Fry the leek for 4–5 minutes until soft and then add the garlic, cooking for a further 2 minutes. Pour in the pearl barley and stir well until the grains are fully coated in the oil. Add the white wine and allow it to bubble and reduce until all of the liquid has been absorbed. Add the chicken stock and salt, stir well and cover, leaving to cook for 35–40 minutes.

INGREDIENTS:

FOR THE RISOTTO:

1 tbsp olive oil

1 leek, halved lengthways and
finely sliced

1 garlic clove, crushed

300g pearl barley

200ml white wine

1 litre good-quality
chicken stock

a large handful of freshly grated
Parmesan cheese

1 tbsp butter

1 tbsp finely chopped
flat-leaf parsley

sea salt

METHOD CONTINUED:

When the chicken has cooked, remove from the oven and transfer onto a plate to rest.

Transfer the vegetables in the baking tray and the chicken juices into a saucepan, place over a high heat, grab a potato masher and mash all of the vegetables and juices together in the saucepan. Allow the vegetables to bubble away in the chicken juices, mashing as you go. Add the plain flour and stir until it starts to thicken. Add the red wine and allow to bubble, stirring constantly, and then add the stock and honey. Give it a good stir and turn down to a simmer, allowing all of the flavours to infuse.

Check the pearl barley is cooked; you're looking for it to be soft but still with a bit of bite. Add the Parmesan, butter and parsley to the pan, give it a good stir and remove from the heat. Pop the lid back on and set aside for a few minutes.

Pop a sieve over a large bowl and carefully strain the gravy. Carve the chicken.

To serve, spoon a ladle of risotto into a bowl, top with chicken and drown in gravy. For a green kick, add a bundle of peppery watercress on top of the chicken and eat straightaway.

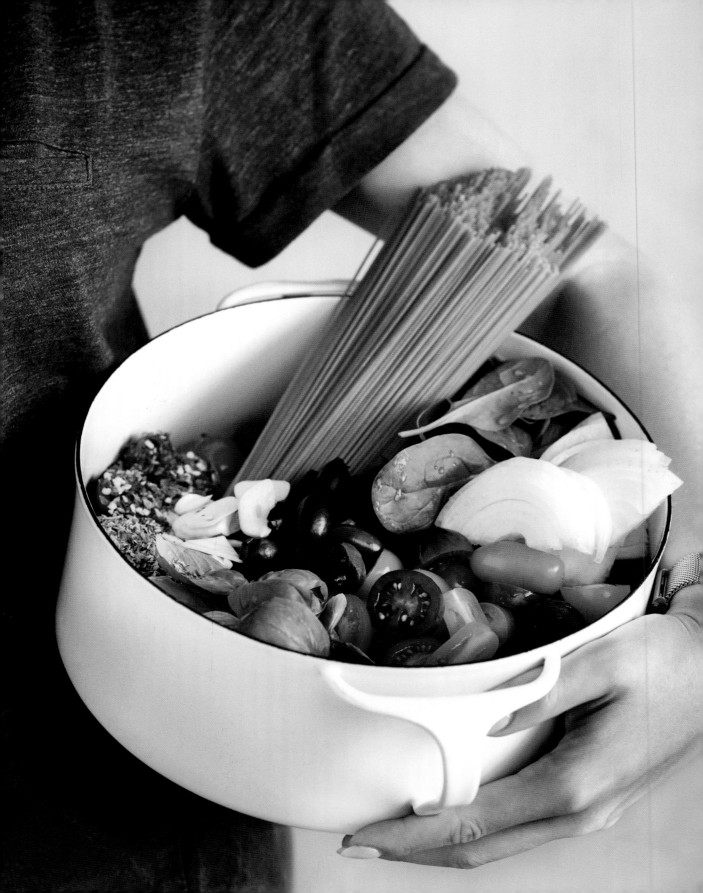

ONE-POT SPELT SPAGHETTI

This dish has saved me on many occasions. Impromptu guests, late-night dinners, hangovers – you name it. Pop it all in a pan, and in 15 minutes you'll have a delicious meal with little effort or work.

INGREDIENTS:

500g dried spelt spaghetti
(wheat pasta is fine here if you
prefer)
500g cherry tomatoes, chopped
(see if you can find them in
different colours)
1 onion, thinly sliced
a large handful of fresh spinach
2 garlic cloves, thinly sliced
a handful of black olives
3 sprigs of fresh basil
4 tbsp olive oil
1 tbsp dried oregano
½ tsp chilli flakes
1 litre hot vegetable stock
sea salt and freshly ground
black pepper

TO SERVE:

a handful of Parmesan cheese,
freshly grated

METHOD:

Place all of the ingredients in a large saucepan and cover with 400ml cold water. Place a lid on and bring to the boil.

Remove the lid, reduce the heat to a simmer and cook for 10 minutes, stirring occasionally until all of the water has evaporated and you're left with a silky sauce.

Serve straight away with lashings of Parmesan cheese.

FRIED CHICKEN THIGHS
WITH HOMEMADE SWEET CHILLI JAM

A nostalgic nod to my favourite teenage comfort food growing up. This version is slightly more sophisticated as a supper with an Asian twist. Serve with green salad, or flash-fried broccoli florets, courgette slices, and toasted cashews with a dash of soy sauce.

INGREDIENTS:

100g cornflour
100g plain flour
4 boneless, skinless chicken thighs
2 eggs, beaten
vegetable oil, for deep-frying
sea salt and freshly ground black pepper

TO SERVE:

Sweet Chilli Jam (page 194)
green salad leaves

METHOD:

In a bowl combine the flours and season with salt and pepper.

Trim off any excess fat from the chicken thighs. One by one, cover the chicken thighs with the seasoned flour, then dip in the beaten egg and then cover again in the flour, creating a thick crust.

Place a heavy-based pan over a medium–high heat and fill with enough vegetable oil to come up to about 4cm. Check to see if the oil is hot enough by dropping a pinch of flour into the oil; if it sizzles, it's hot enough. Fry the chicken thighs two at a time until golden and crisp.

Remove and drain on kitchen paper. When cool enough to handle, slice each thigh into three.

Serve with a crisp green salad and Sweet Chilli Jam (p 194).

THE ULTIMATE MAC AND CHEESE

SERVES

4

Cheese, cheese, more cheese and pasta. Dairy and gluten – HURRAH! We only live once, and life is too short not to enjoy my ultimate mac and cheese. There are no rules with this – whatever cheese you have, whatever's your favourite, throw it in. Stick to the measurements but – as a suggestion – it's really good with a bit of Stilton, Red Leicester or just made entirely out of Cheddar, it really doesn't matter. Serve with a crisp and tangy side salad and a glass of white wine. Heavenly.

INGREDIENTS:

300g dried macaroni

2 tbsp butter

3 tbsp plain flour

500ml whole milk

100g mature Cheddar, grated

100g Gruyère, grated

50g mozzarella, grated

50g Parmesan, grated

1 tbsp wholegrain mustard

50g breadcrumbs

sea salt and freshly ground black pepper

METHOD:

Preheat the oven to 200°C/180°C fan/ Gas mark 6.

Bring a large pan of salted water to the boil and cook the macaroni for 2 minutes less than the packet instructions.

Meanwhile, make the cheese sauce. Melt the butter in a large pan over a medium heat. Sprinkle in the flour and stir for 1 minute.

Slowly pour in the milk, whisking continuously, until you have a smooth sauce with no lumps. Reduce the heat and add the cheeses, mustard and salt and pepper and stir until the cheeses have melted and everything is combined.

Drain the macaroni and tumble it into the cheese sauce. Stir carefully to combine and then pour out into a 20cm ovenproof dish. Cover with breadcrumbs and cook in the oven for 20–25 minutes until golden brown. Allow to rest for a few minutes before dishing up.

MIKE'S PAELLA

This paella was one of the first things Mike ever made for me and he's been making it for me ever since. It's one of the best paellas I've ever had and so, in honour of its greatness, I'm sharing it with you. This recipe works best if you have a paella pan. If not, use the biggest shallow frying pan you have.

INGREDIENTS:

olive oil
4 chicken thighs, cut in half
200g chorizo, cut into thick chunks
1 large white onion, finely chopped
2 garlic cloves, finely chopped
1 red pepper, core removed and roughly chopped
500g Spanish short grain paella rice
½ tsp chilli flakes
2 tsp paprika
150ml dry white wine
1 litre good-quality chicken stock
a good pinch saffron
approximately 20 mussels, scrubbed and de-bearded
3 large tomatoes, chopped
100g frozen peas
15 shell-on jumbo king prawns
150g squid, cleaned and cut into rings
sea salt and freshly ground black pepper

TO SERVE:

a large handful of flat-leaf parsley
1 lemon, cut into wedges

METHOD:

Heat a good glug of olive oil in a paella dish or heavy-based saucepan over a medium–high heat, then fry the chicken thighs until browned all over. Set aside. Add the chorizo to the pan and cook until lightly browned.

Add the onion, half of the garlic and the pepper and cook for a few minutes until soft. Pour in the rice and stir until all the grains are coated. Add the chilli flakes, paprika, salt and pepper and wine and give it a good stir. Once it's bubbling, pour in the chicken stock, scatter in the saffron and add the chicken thighs back into the pan and cook on a medium heat for 10–12 minutes.

Reduce the heat and push the mussels into the rice with the join facing down so that the shells open upwards. Cover with the tomatoes and cook for 5 minutes. Add the peas and cook for a further 5 minutes.

Heat the remaining garlic in some oil in a small frying pan on a medium heat and then add the prawns. Fry for a few minutes until they've turned pink, then add them to the paella. Add the squid into the same pan and cook for a couple of minutes, adding to the paella once done.

Sprinkle over the chopped parsley and serve immediately with lemon wedges.

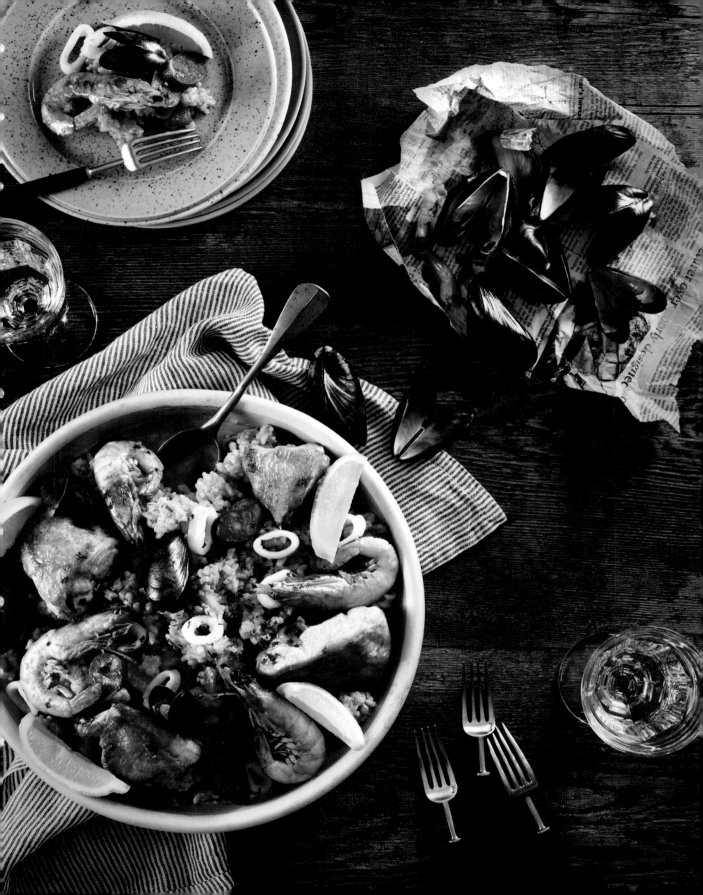

LEMON AND PROSCIUTTO FETTUCCINI

SERVES
2

Easy-peasy lemon squeezy – quite literally. I eat this dish on Christmas Eve, once all the food prep is done and I want an easy, delicious and comforting bowl of pasta, but it's great throughout the year. Team with a crisp green salad during the summer, or with some homemade garlic bread for the colder months.

INGREDIENTS:

4 slices prosciutto

1 tbsp butter

1 garlic clove, crushed

1 tbsp plain flour

200ml chicken stock

a large handful of freshly grated Parmesan cheese, plus extra for serving

zest and juice of ½ unwaxed lemon

200g fresh fettuccini

sea salt and freshly ground black pepper

METHOD:

Place a heavy-based pan over a medium heat and fry the prosciutto for a couple of minutes until crisp. Remove and drain on kitchen paper.

In the same pan, melt the butter and fry the garlic for a minute until it starts to brown. Add the flour and stir to form a paste. Continue to cook for a minute or two, stirring constantly.

Slowly add the chicken stock, stirring vigorously, until you have a loose, smooth sauce. Remove from the heat, add the Parmesan, lemon zest and juice and a pinch of salt and pepper, then stir well. Keep warm.

Bring a pan of salted water to the boil and cook the fettuccini as per the packet instructions.

Once al dente, pour over the sauce and mix well. Crumble over the prosciutto and serve immediately with extra Parmesan.

COQ AU VIN PIE

SERVES
4

Coq au Vin in a pie. I mean, I don't want to boast or anything, but why is this not a thing?! Do this and you won't look back, I promise you. Chicken cooked in a deliciously rich red wine gravy topped with flaky puff pastry? A match made in heaven.

INGREDIENTS:

90g butter
3 large skinless chicken breasts, halved
150g pancetta or bacon lardons
1 medium onion, roughly chopped
1 large carrot, peeled and roughly chopped
2 celery sticks, roughly chopped
2 garlic cloves, finely chopped
2 tbsp plain flour
1 bottle red wine
2 bay leaves
12 shallots, peeled and halved
200g chestnut mushrooms, left whole or halved if large
1 tsp Marmite
1 x 375g pack ready-rolled puff pastry
1 egg, beaten
sea salt and freshly ground black pepper

METHOD:

Preheat the oven to 200°C/180°C fan/Gas mark 6.

Heat 50g butter in a heavy-based pan, placed over a medium-high heat. Add the chicken breasts and sear until golden brown. Remove from the pan and set aside.

In the same pan, fry the pancetta until it starts to brown. Remove from the pan and drain on kitchen paper.

Add the onions, carrot, celery and garlic to the oil and cook for a few minutes until soft.

Add the flour and continue to cook for a couple of minutes, stirring until everything is coated. Pour in the wine and bring to the boil. Reduce to a simmer, then add the bay leaves and salt and pepper.

In a small pan, heat the remaining butter over a high heat and fry the shallots and mushrooms until browned. Transfer to the pan of wine and vegetables and add the Marmite. Return the chicken and pancetta to the pan and stir well. Cover and cook in the oven for 40 minutes.

When the cooking time is up, remove the pan from the oven. Lift the chicken breasts out and roughly shred, before returning to the pan. Set aside to cool.

Spoon the cooled coq au vin into a 28cm pie dish, evening out with the back of a spoon. Unroll the pastry over the dish, pressing the pastry down into the corners and folding any excess pastry under the rim – we're going for a rustic look, so the more pastry, the better!

Score the pastry lid on the diagonal, brush with more egg wash and bake in the oven for 20–25 minutes until the pastry is golden brown.

JERK AND RIOJA LAMB SHANKS
WITH RICE AND PEAS

SERVES

4

I created this recipe when a friend came over for dinner. Asked what he liked to eat, he said Caribbean food and lamb… OK, what the heck do I do with that? From that experimental journey came this dish, one I now crave in the colder months, and which is loved by friends and always cooked on request for my father's birthday.

INGREDIENTS:

FOR THE MARINADE:

100ml dark rum

100ml ginger beer

zest and juice of 1 orange

1 tbsp jerk seasoning

1 cinnamon stick, broken in half

1 tsp allspice

1 large red chilli, cut in half

a sprig of fresh thyme

a few garlic cloves

4 lamb shanks

METHOD:

Pop all of the marinade ingredients in a large bowl and stir well.

Pierce the lamb shanks with a knife and rub all over with the marinade. Allow the lamb shanks to marinate in the fridge overnight.

The following day, preheat the oven to 150°C/130°C fan/Gas mark 2.

Heat, a glug of olive oil in a heavy-based pan placed over a high heat. (Ensure the pan isn't too big; you want the lamb shanks to fit snugly in the pan.)

Remove the lamb shanks from the marinade and fry until browned on all sides. Remove from the pan and set aside. Add the onion, garlic and carrots and stir well. Pour in the wine and deglaze the pan, getting all the delicious, sticky cooking juices up from the bottom of the pan. Pop the lamb shanks back in the pan and add the balsamic vinegar and 100ml water then crumble in the stock cube.

Strain the marinade and add three-quarters of it to the pan.

Bring to the boil, then cover and cook on the middle of the oven for 3 hours, turning the shanks half way through.

INGREDIENTS:

FOR THE SAUCE:

olive oil

1 onion, quartered

2 garlic cloves, finely chopped

2 carrots, peeled and chopped
into thick chunks

200ml red wine

2 tbsp balsamic vinegar

1 lamb stock cube

sea salt and freshly ground
pepper

FOR THE RICE
AND PEAS:

1 x 400g tin coconut milk

1 tin measurement
chicken stock

1 tin measurement white rice

a sprig of thyme

½ tsp allspice

1 x 400g tin kidney beans,
drained

butter

METHOD CONTINUED:

Once the shanks are cooked, carefully remove them from the pan and cover with foil to keep warm.

Place a pan over a medium–high heat and add the coconut milk. Fill the empty tin with rice and add to the pan and then repeat with the chicken stock. This is the perfect ratio of rice for 4 hungry people. Bring to the boil, add the thyme and allspice, cover and leave on a low simmer for 15 minutes. If at any time it needs more water, just add a splash. Just before the end of cooking, add the kidney beans and a knob of butter then put the lid back on.

Meanwhile, place the lamb cooking pan over a medium–high heat and reduce the sauce for 10–15 minutes. You're looking for a gravy consistency that's lovely and glossy. Check the seasoning.

Serve the lamb shanks covered with the sauce poured over and the rice and peas on the side.

ASIAN BEEF LETTUCE CUPS

SERVES
2

For those of you who always order crispy shredded chilli beef for your Chinese takeaway – I understand. But however wonderfully gluttonous a takeaway can be, it sometimes gets a bit much – for the waistline and for the wallet. So, in times of need and without stretching the bank balance, I have the perfect solution. These crispy beef cups are delicious and really hit the spot. Nestled into lettuce cups with cucumber ribbons, toasted cashews, spring onion and chilli, these are a delicious take on the classic and, perhaps, even better.

INGREDIENTS:

4 tbsp cornflour
500g sirloin steak, bashed out to a 5mm thickness and sliced into strips
vegetable oil, for deep-frying
sea salt and freshly ground black pepper

FOR THE CHILLI SAUCE:

100ml sweet chilli sauce
zest and juice of 1 orange
juice of 1 lime
2 tbsp dark soy sauce
1 tsp fish sauce

TO SERVE:

mini Cos or Little Gem lettuce leaves
1 cucumber cut into ribbons
2 tbsp crushed toasted cashews (optional)
1 spring onion, finely sliced
1 red chilli, finely sliced

METHOD:

To make the sauce, place a pan over a medium–high heat and add the sweet chilli sauce, orange juice and zest, lime juice, dark soy and fish sauce. Bring to the boil and then reduce the heat to a simmer until the sauce becomes glossy and sticky. Set aside while you fry the beef.

Put 2 tablespoons cornflour in a bowl and season with salt and pepper. Add the beef strips and toss to coat.

Half-fill a heavy-based pan with vegetable oil and place on a medium heat. Drop a pinch of cornflour into the oil; when it starts to bubble on the surface, the oil is hot enough.

Carefully add the beef strips to the pan and fry for a couple of minutes until they are pale golden. Remove from the pan with a slotted spoon and set aside.

Add the remaining 2 tablespoons cornflour to a clean bowl. Add the cooked beef and toss to coat once more.

Return the beef strips to the pan, increasing the heat a little, and fry until golden brown.

Turn off the heat and, using a slotted spoon, remove the beef from the pan and drain on kitchen paper before coating in the chilli sauce.

To serve, lay the lettuce leaves over a platter and fill each one with cucumber ribbons, the crispy chilli beef, toasted cashews (if using), spring onion and chilli.

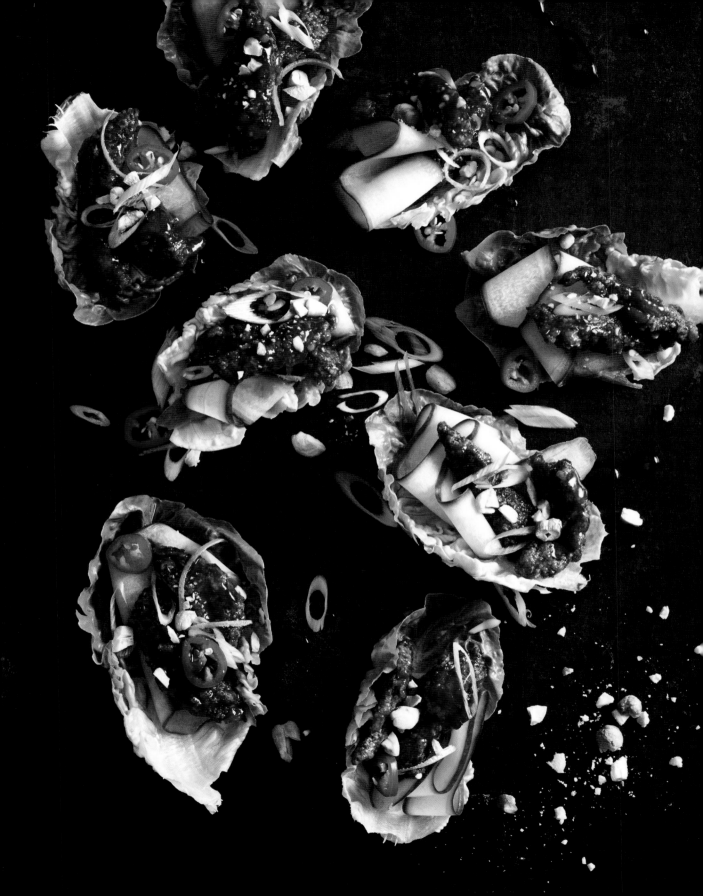

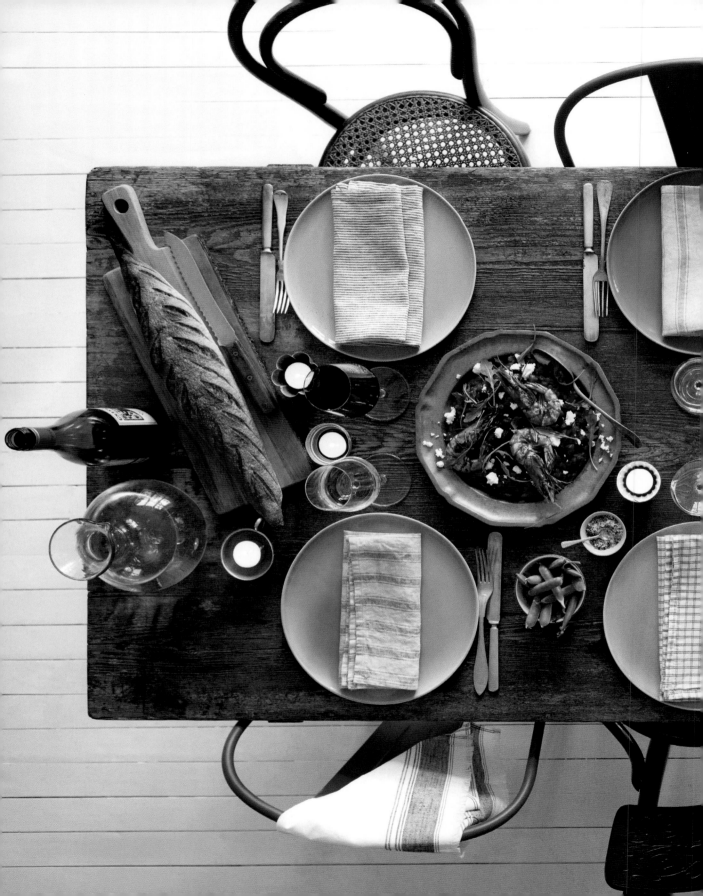

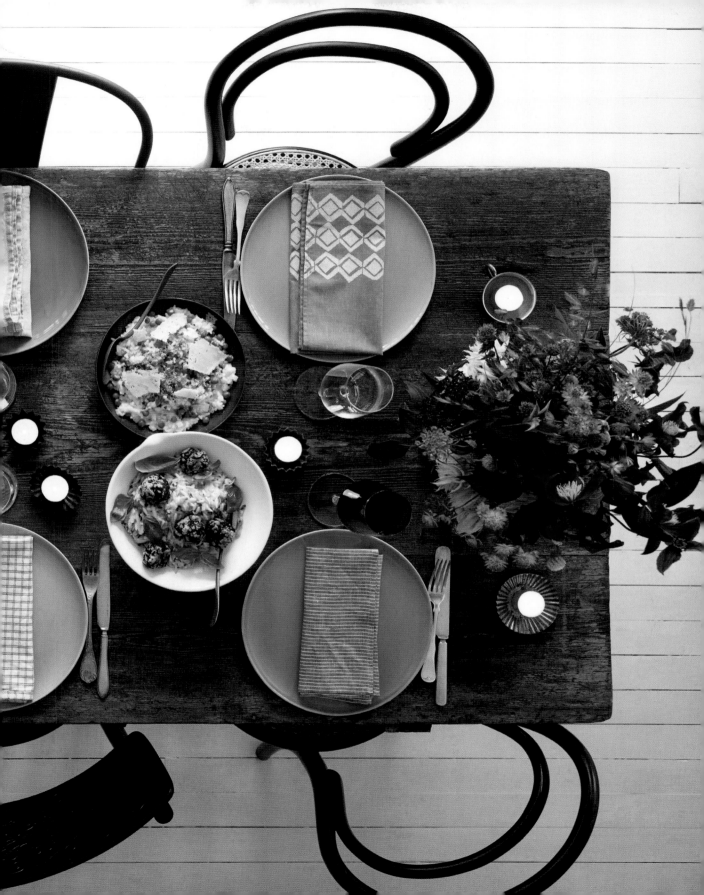

SICILIAN MACKEREL WITH CAPERS, PINE NUTS AND SULTANAS

This is an easy, delicious recipe with Sicilian ingredients. Sweet sultanas and salty capers work really well together, creating a dish with lots of wonderfully contrasting but harmonising flavours. Serve with a green salad in the summer or with new potatoes and greens in the winter.

SERVES
4

INGREDIENTS:

1 tbsp sultanas

olive oil

½ red onion, thinly sliced

4 mackerel fillets

2 tbsp red wine vinegar

1 tsp balsamic vinegar

1 tsp honey

1 tbsp capers

1 tbsp pine nuts, toasted

a few sprigs of fresh dill

extra-virgin olive oil

sea salt and freshly ground black pepper

TO SERVE:

new potatoes, boiled

a green salad

METHOD:

Boil the kettle and pour enough water over the sultanas to cover them.

Heat a glug of olive oil in a pan placed over a medium heat, then cook the onion for a few minutes until soft.

Place a griddle pan over a high heat. Brush the skin of the mackerel fillets with olive oil and season with salt. Place skin-side down and cook for 3 minutes. Turn over the fish and cook for a further minute.

Meanwhile, drain the sultanas and add to the onions along with the vinegars, honey and capers. Stir well. Add the pine nuts and dill, season with a little salt and pepper and a good glug of extra-virgin olive oil.

To serve, pour the sauce on a platter and top with the fish. Finish with a sprinkling of dill.

Serve with boiled new potatoes or a green salad.

AUBERGINE LASAGNE

SERVES

4

When you want the comfort of a lasagne but without all the meat and stodge, this is the solution. Based on a classic Melanzane alla Parmigiana, this is a delicious and hearty Italian dish. The aubergine soaks up all of the flavours and adds a wonderful texture to the dish. This is how I like to make mine, and how I was taught by someone's *nonna* once upon a time. You'll need a baking dish about 30cm x 20cm for this one.

INGREDIENTS:

2 aubergines, thinly sliced
olive oil
1 onion, finely chopped
2 garlic cloves,
finely chopped
1 carrot, finely chopped
1 celery stick, finely chopped
1 tsp dried oregano
1 tsp dried thyme
1 tsp dried basil
1 x 700g jar passata
100ml red wine
1 tsp caster sugar
2 balls of fresh mozzarella,
shredded
plenty of freshly grated
Parmesan cheese
sea salt and freshly ground
black pepper

TO SERVE:

fresh basil leaves

METHOD:

Sprinkle the aubergine with salt and sandwich the slices between a kitchen towel, patting them down to soak up any excess moisture.

Place a griddle pan over a high heat, add the aubergine slices and cook until they're slightly soft and have black char marks over them. Remove from the pan and set aside.

In a large pan, heat a little olive oil over a medium heat and add the onion, garlic, carrot and celery. Cook for 7–10 minutes until soft.

Add the herbs and pour in the passata. Pour the wine into the empty passata jar and shake well to remove any leftover tomato sauce and add to the pan. Bring to the boil, then reduce the heat. Add the sugar, season well with salt and pepper and allow to simmer for 35–40 minutes until thick and rich.

Preheat the oven to 200°C/180°C fan/Gas mark 6.

To assemble the lasagne, spoon a ladle-full of tomato sauce over the bottom of the baking dish. Add a layer of aubergine slices and cover with a ladle of sauce and then a third of the shredded mozzarella and repeat, leaving some mozzarella for the top layer.

Scatter the top with freshly grated Parmesan and bake for 25–30 minutes. Scatter with fresh basil and serve.

SWEET AND STICKY PORK RIBS

A hit with all my friends, especially the guys, these are the perfect ribs. They're easy to make and absolutely packed with flavour, so prepare to be asked for seconds and thirds.

SERVES
4

INGREDIENTS:

2 racks of pork ribs,
approximately 700g each
2 tbsp Chinese five spice
1 tsp toasted sesame oil
2 tbsp light soy sauce
2 tbsp honey
1 tbsp fish sauce
juice of ½ large orange
juice of 1 lime
1 spring onion, finely sliced
1 red chilli, finely sliced

METHOD:

Preheat the oven to 200°C/180°C fan/Gas mark 6.

Rub the pork ribs all over with the Chinese five spice and pop in a high rimmed baking tray. Cook the ribs on the middle shelf of the oven for 45 minutes.

To make the sauce, combine the toasted sesame oil, soy sauce, honey, fish sauce, orange and lime juice and 2 tablespoons water in a bowl.

Remove the ribs from the oven and decrease the temperature to 180°C/160°F fan/Gas mark 4. Spoon a third of the sauce over the ribs and return to the oven for another 45 minutes.

When the ribs are nearly ready, put the remaining sauce in a small pan placed over a medium–high heat. Reduce until the sauce is thickened and sticky.

Remove the ribs from the oven and slather in the sticky sauce, scatter with the spring onion and chilli and serve immediately.

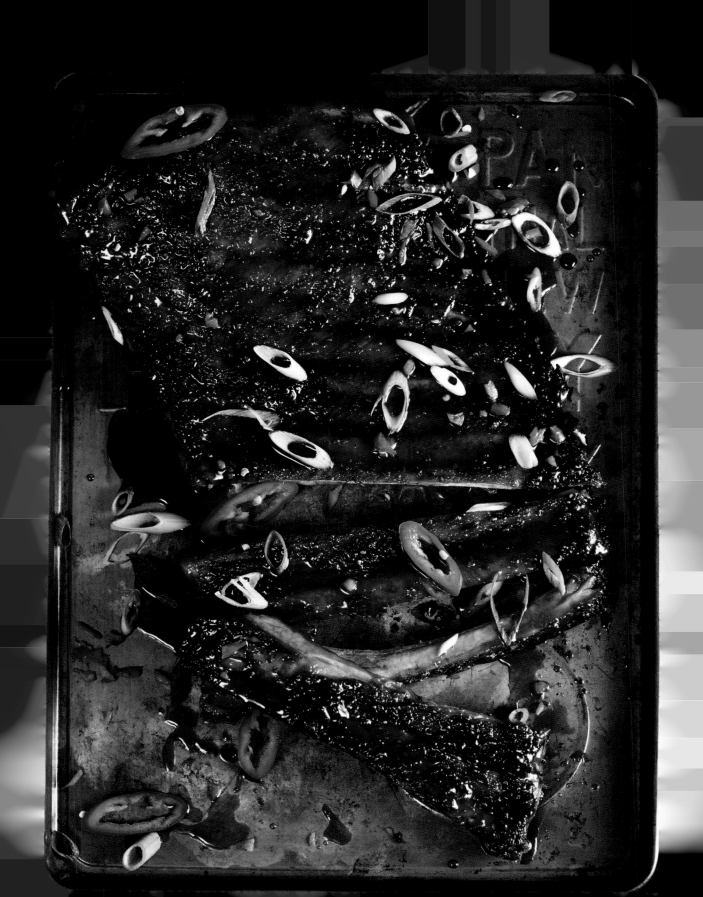

SALMON AND BROWN RICE PATTIES
WITH WATERCRESS AND LIME SOURED CREAM

This recipe came from one of those "there's no food in the cupboard" days. I always have a bag of microwavable rice available; they're a life saver. One time, I also had some leftover salmon in the fridge but no vegetables to go with it, so I created this recipe. The texture might not be to everyone's taste – the consistency is similar to a Thai fish cake though with rice – but I urge you to try it before you decide. Team with tangy lime-infused soured cream and fresh watercress; it's a nourishing, light and healthy dinner.

INGREDIENTS:

2 skinless, salmon fillets
1 x 250g packet
microwavable brown rice,
cooked
zest and juice of 1 lime
a small handful of coriander
leaves, chopped
1 tbsp cream cheese
olive oil
4 tbsp soured cream
a handful of watercress
sea salt and freshly ground
black pepper

METHOD:

In a food processor, pulse the salmon fillets with half of the brown rice until it forms a chunky paste and tip into a bowl.

Add the remaining brown rice, half of the lime juice and zest, coriander and cream cheese. Season with salt and pepper and mix well. Using your hands, form into 4 patties.

Place a non-stick pan over a medium heat and add a little olive oil. Fry the patties for a few minutes on each side until golden brown and cooked through.

Mix the soured cream with the remaining lime zest and juice and season well with salt and pepper.

Serve the patties with a handful of fresh watercress and a dollop of the lime soured cream on the side.

MOROCCAN SHEPHERD'S PIE

While filming last year, I had one of the best-ever catered lunches. The cooks created a Moroccan-style shepherd's pie with purple sweet potato. Everyone who tried it went for seconds (or, in my case, thirds). I've tried to replicate it, and I hope I've done them proud! This is a sweet and aromatic take on a classic dish that will get people talking.

INGREDIENTS:

500g lamb mince
1 tbsp olive oil
1 large red onion,
finely chopped
2 garlic cloves,
finely chopped
2 celery sticks,
finely chopped
2 carrots, finely chopped
1 tsp cumin
1 tsp paprika
1 tsp cinnamon
1 tsp chilli powder
1 x 400g tin cherry tomatoes
a handful of dried apricots,
roughly chopped
1 tsp honey
800g sweet potatoes
butter
1 tbsp finely chopped
flat-leaf parsley
sea salt and freshly ground
black pepper

METHOD:

Preheat the oven to 200°C/180°C fan/Gas mark 6.

Heat the oil in a heavy-based pan set over a medium heat. Fry the lamb until browned all over. Set aside.

Reduce the heat and add the onion, garlic, celery and carrot and cook for 10 minutes until soft. Add the spices and continue to cook for a couple of minutes.

Return the lamb back into the pan along with the tinned tomatoes, apricots, honey and 50ml water. Season with a good pinch of salt and pepper and bring to the boil. Cover with the lid and reduce the heat to a simmer for 1 hour.

The sauce should have thickened by now, but if it's still a little watery, take off the lid and simmer for another 10 minutes. Remove from the heat and set aside while you prepare the sweet potatoes.

Peel the sweet potatoes and chop into large chunks. Cook in boiling salted water for about 15 minutes until very soft. Drain and add a knob of butter.

Using a potato masher, mash the potatoes until smooth, but don't worry too much about getting it perfectly smooth, it's quite nice rustic.

Transfer the lamb to an ovenproof casserole dish and spread the mashed potato over the top.

Bake for 25–30 minutes until the sweet potato is crispy around the edges.

Scatter with chopped parsley and serve.

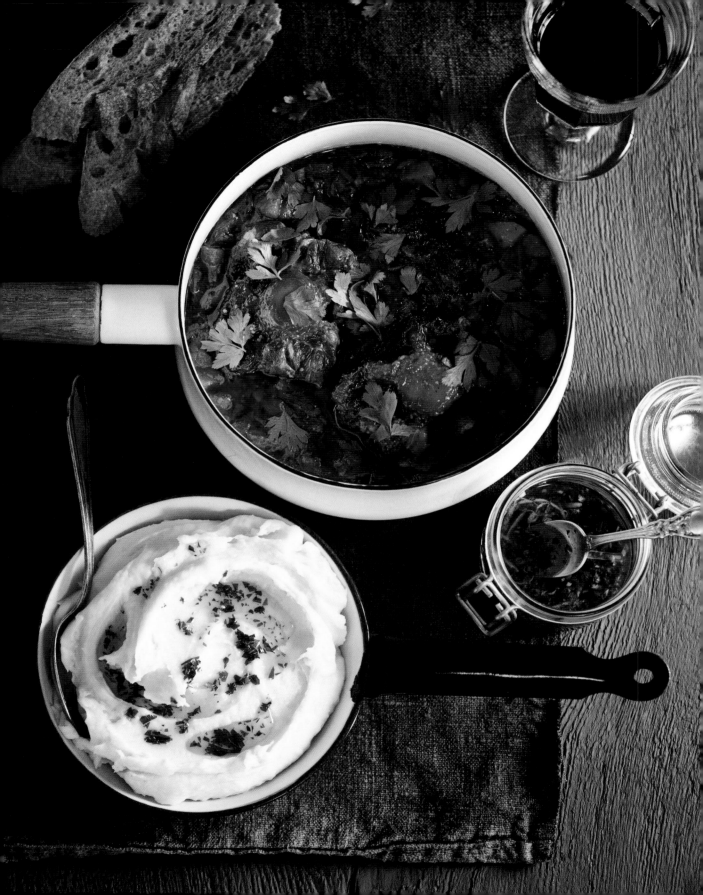

SLOW-COOKED OXTAIL RAGU
WITH PARMESAN MASH AND GREMOLATA OIL

SERVES
4

A few years ago, I learnt to cook a dish with oxtail and was hooked. For those who wouldn't know what to do with oxtail or who think it's old-fashioned, trust me on this one. You won't look back. When slow-cooked for hours, it releases the sweetest and most delicious flavor, one you'll never get from steak. My advice? Make this a day ahead, and reheat again the following day for even more flavour. Fish out the bones and shred the meat before serving for a fuss-free dish.

INGREDIENTS:

FOR THE OXTAIL RAGU:

olive oil

1kg oxtail cut into approximately 4–5 thick chunks

butter

2 carrots, peeled and roughly chopped

1 onion, roughly chopped

2 garlic cloves, finely chopped

2 celery sticks, roughly chopped

200ml red wine

1 x 400g tin cherry tomatoes

1 tbsp wholegrain mustard

1 tbsp tomato purée

1 tbsp Worcestershire sauce

1 litre good-quality beef stock

sea salt and freshly ground black pepper

METHOD:

Preheat the oven to 150°C/130°C fan/Gas mark 2.

Place a heavy-based pan over a high heat and add a glug of olive oil. Season the oxtail with salt and pepper and cook for a few minutes until browned on all sides. Remove from the pan and set aside.

Add a knob of butter and throw in the carrots, onion, garlic and celery. Cook for 5 minutes until soft, then pour in the wine to deglaze the pan.

Add the cherry tomatoes, mustard, tomato purée, Worcestershire sauce and beef stock and bring to the boil. Return the oxtail to the pan, cover with a lid and cook on the middle shelf of the oven for 4 hours.

To make the mash, peel the potatoes and cut into chunks. Boil the potatoes in salted water for 15 minutes or until soft. Drain, transfer back to the pan and mash together with the butter, Parmesan and a good pinch of salt and pepper.

continued overleaf

SLOW-COOKED OXTAIL RAGU
WITH PARMESAN MASH AND GREMOLATA OIL
CONT...

INGREDIENTS:

FOR THE PARMESAN MASH:

500g Maris Piper potatoes
50g butter
a large handful of freshly grated
Parmesan cheese
sea salt and freshly ground
black pepper

FOR THE GREMOLATA OIL:

½ bunch of flat-leaf parsley,
finely chopped
1 garlic clove, finely chopped
zest of ½ unwaxed lemon
100ml extra-virgin olive oil

METHOD CONTINUED:

Meanwhile, make the gremolata oil. Place the parsley and garlic in a bowl and add the lemon zest. Pour in the extra-virgin olive oil and stir well.

Once the oxtail is cooked, you can serve it whole as it is or shred the meat before serving. As oxtail is quite a fatty cut, I like to shred mine. To do this, simply remove the oxtail from the pan, shred the meat away from the bone and return to the pan. Stir the shredded meat into the ragu and serve with a spoonful of Parmesan mash and a drizzle of gremolata oil.

ONE-POT STICKY SAUSAGE AND THREE-BEAN CASSOULET

In the colder months there's nothing more comforting than a sticky sausage stew. Even better, it's all cooked in one pan. Super-simple to make and low-maintenance on the washing up – good news all round. Leave to bubble away until it's ready – the longer it stays on the hob, the better. This isn't a typical cassoulet, but it's how I like mine. Serve with lots of greens and a hunk of crusty bread.

SERVES
6

INGREDIENTS:

12 good-quality pork sausages
2 x 130g packs cubed pancetta
2 red onions, sliced
2 garlic cloves, finely chopped
300ml red wine
a few sprigs of fresh thyme
a few sprigs of fresh rosemary
1 x 200g tin baked beans
1 x 200g tin haricot beans, drained
1 x 200g tin kidney beans, drained
1 heaped tbsp wholegrain mustard
1 tbsp tomato purée
a squeeze of honey
1 x 400g tin cherry tomatoes
a small loaf of stale bread, such as ciabatta, ripped into large chunks
sea salt and freshly ground black pepper

TO SERVE:

fresh bread

METHOD:

In a large heavy-based pan, fry the sausages until browned on all sides, then remove from the pan and set aside.

Add the pancetta to the pan and cook until browned, then add the onions and garlic and cook for a couple of minutes until soft.

Deglaze the pan by pouring in the wine and then add the herbs, beans, mustard, tomato purée, honey and cherry tomatoes. Season with salt and pepper and bring to the boil. Reduce the heat, return the sausages to the pan and simmer for 15 minutes.

Lay the bread chunks over the cassoulet. Drizzle with olive oil and cook in the oven for 35–40 minutes.

Serve with a hunk of crusty bread to mop up all the juices.

CHICKEN KATSU CURRY BURGERS
WITH PICKLED ASIAN SLAW

SERVES
2

INGREDIENTS:

FOR THE KATSU SAUCE:

1 tbsp vegetable oil
1 onion, roughly chopped
5 garlic cloves, roughly chopped
2 carrots, peeled and grated
2 tbsp plain flour
1 tbsp medium curry powder
1 tsp garam masala
600ml chicken stock
1 tbsp honey
1 tbsp soy sauce

FOR THE CHICKEN BURGERS:

2 free-range chicken breasts
2 tbsp plain flour
1 egg, beaten
4 tbsp panko breadcrumbs
200ml vegetable oil, for frying
small handful coriander and shredded spring onions, to serve
2 brioche burger buns, cut in half lengthways

FOR THE PICKLED ASIAN SLAW:

1 carrot, peeled into ribbons or julienned
¼ red cabbage, shredded
1 pak choi, shredded
2 spring onions, finely sliced
2 tbsp rice wine vinegar or malt vinegar
2 tbsp soy sauce
1 tsp soft brown sugar
1 tsp salt

This one is a no-brainer for me: two of my favourite things – katsu curry and chicken burger – combined. Add as much heat to the katsu sauce as you want in the shape of the garam masala. I like the contrast of the heat and the tangy pickled slaw. Alternatively, make double the slaw and serve on the side.

METHOD:

To make the sauce, heat the vegetable oil in a pan placed over a medium–high heat. Add the onion, garlic and grated carrot and cook for a few minutes until soft. Add the flour, curry powder and garam masala and stir until fully coated.

Slowly pour in the chicken stock, whisking continuously to prevent any lumps forming. Add the honey and soy sauce and simmer for 15–20 minutes until thick but still pourable. Set aside on a low heat.

To make the chicken burgers, coat the chicken breasts with flour, then the egg and then the panko breadcrumbs.

Heat the vegetable oil in a pan over a medium–high heat and cook the chicken breasts for 5–8 minutes on each side until cooked through.

To make the slaw, combine all the prepped vegetables in a bowl with the vinegar, soy sauce, sugar and salt. Stir well.

To assemble the burgers, place a heap of the Asian pickled slaw on the bottom half of the brioche bun, top with the chicken breast, spoon over the sauce and top with coriander and shredded spring onions.

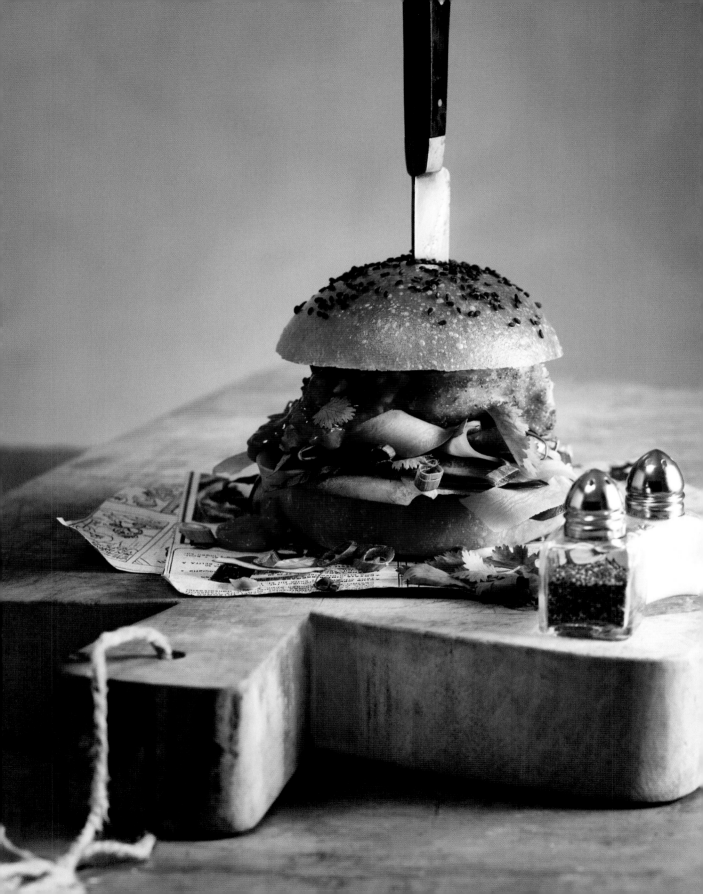

CREAMY SAFFRON AND PROSECCO MUSSELS

SERVES
4

Saffron and prosecco – it doesn't get much better than that now, does it? I've always been a fan of moules marinière, and this recipe mixes things up. Not only does it taste indulgent and wonderful, but the saffron creates the most beautiful-coloured soupy sauce, making it a fantastic centrepiece.

INGREDIENTS:

olive oil
1 leek, halved lengthways and sliced
1 garlic clove, thinly sliced
300ml Prosecco
1 pinch of saffron
3kg fresh mussels, de-bearded, discarding any that don't close with a gentle tap
50ml double cream
1 tbsp finely chopped flat-leaf parsley
sea salt and freshly ground black pepper

TO SERVE:

any fresh bread of your choice

METHOD:

Pour a glug of olive oil in a heavy-based pan placed over a medium–high heat. Add the leek and cook for a few minutes until soft. Add the garlic and cook for a couple more minutes, then pour in the Prosecco, sprinkle in the saffron and bring to the boil.

Carefully tip in the mussels, cover and reduce the heat and cook for 3–4 minutes or until the mussels have opened.

Remove from the heat and discard any mussels that haven't opened.

Pour in the double cream, season with salt and pepper and sprinkle over the chopped parsley. Serve immediately with fresh bread.

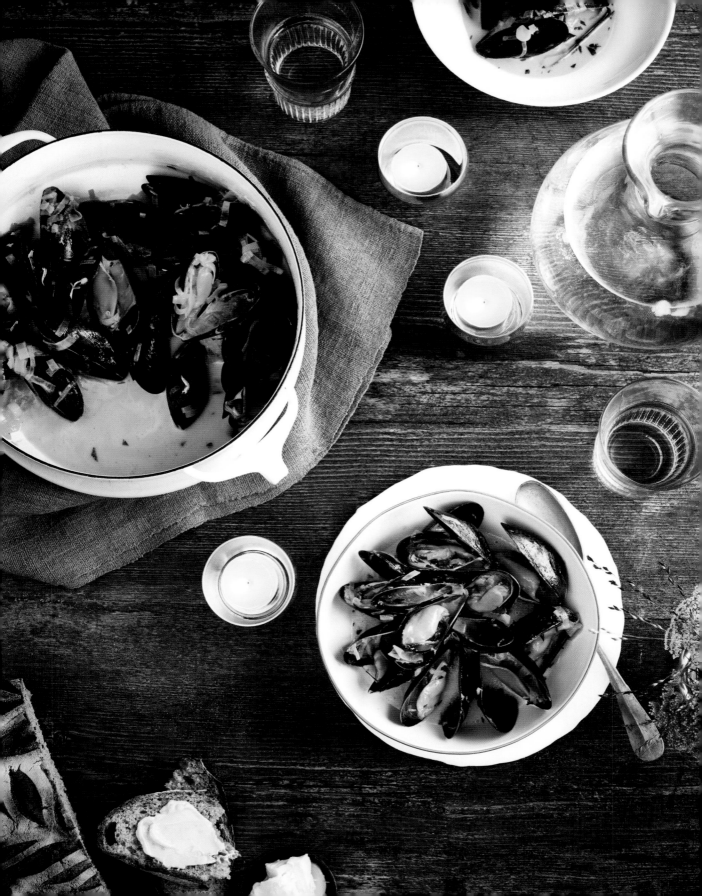

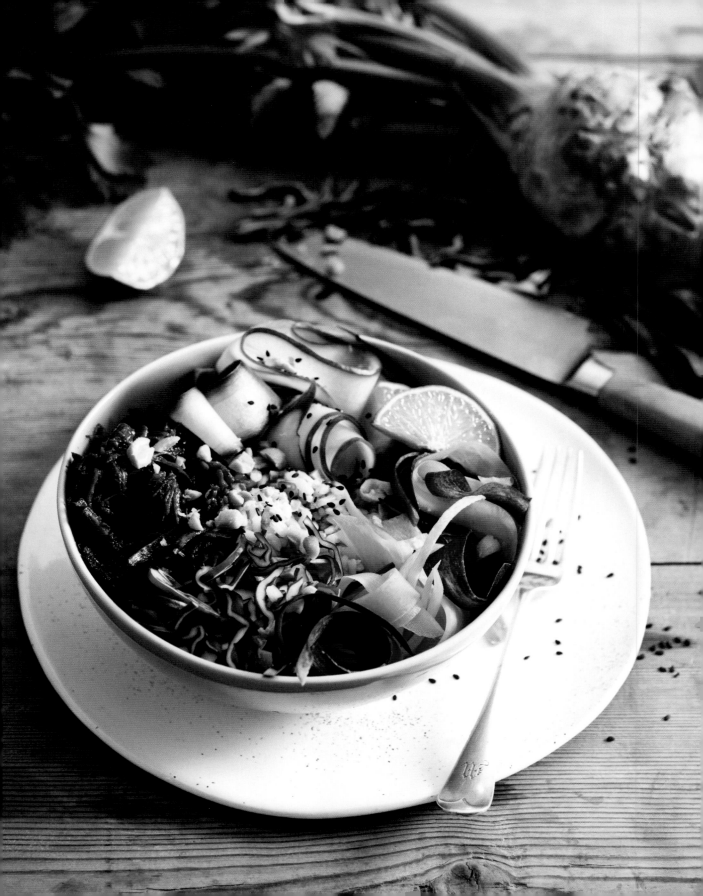

HONEY GARLIC SHREDDED BEEF AND BROWN RICE BOWLS

SERVES
3 – 4

Rice bowls are one of my weekday staples. We usually have beef in the freezer, so I'll whip it out in the morning to let it defrost, then come dinnertime, it's easy to heat and shred the beef and assemble with fresh salad and rice to make a bowl. Anything goes in this recipe: use whatever salad you have, just shred it all up. This is how I like to eat mine.

INGREDIENTS:

1 tbsp vegetable oil

500g lean casserole steak

1 celery stick, diced

1 carrot, diced

1 onion, diced

2 garlic gloves, finely chopped

200ml chicken stock

50ml dark soy sauce

1 tsp fish sauce

3 tbsp honey

2 x 250g packet microwavable brown rice

1 cucumber, peeled into ribbons

2 carrots shredded or peeled into ribbons

¼ red cabbage, shredded

1 lime, quartered

1 tbsp salted peanuts, crushed

METHOD:

Preheat the oven to 150°C/130°C fan/Gas mark 2.

Heat the oil in an ovenproof non-stick pan, then sear the steak over a high heat. Once browned on all sides remove from the pan and set aside.

Reduce the heat and throw in the celery, carrot, onion and garlic and cook for 5 minutes until soft. Return the steak to the pan and add the chicken stock, soy sauce, fish sauce and honey. Bring to the boil, reduce to a simmer and pop in the oven for two hours.

Take the pan out of the oven and remove the meat. If there's still a lot of liquid in the pan, place over a medium–high heat to reduce for a few minutes.

Shred the meat with two forks, then return to the pan and stir well.

Cook the rice as per the packet instructions.

To assemble the bowls, pour the rice into the centre of the bowl and surround with the cucumber ribbons, carrots, red cabbage, lime wedges and crushed peanuts.

Serve immediately.

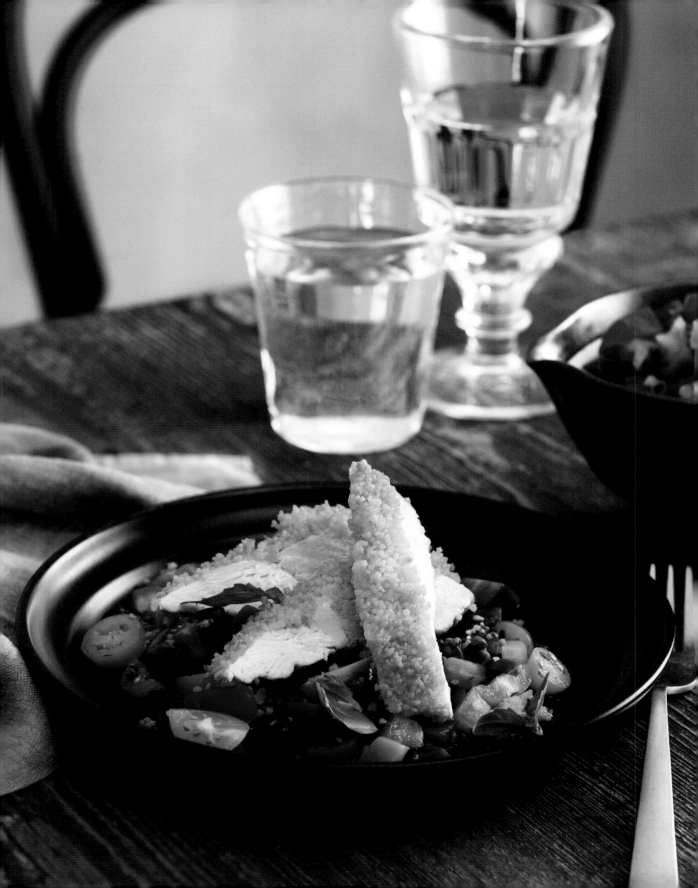

COUSCOUS-CRUSTED CHICKEN
WITH CHUNKY PUTTANESCA

SERVES
2

A deceptively simple dish. It's fresh, flavoursome and takes hardly any effort. When tomatoes are in season try to get as many different varieties as you can; large, small, long, green, yellow, orange and red, fluted or fat – they each have different flavours adding so much freshness to the dish. Don't be put off by the anchovies – they melt down, adding depth of flavour to the dish – but if you really can't stand them leave them out.

INGREDIENTS:

100ml white wine
75g couscous
a good pinch of saffron
2 free-range chicken breasts
1 tbsp plain flour
1 egg, beaten
100g various tomatoes, deseeded and finely chopped
50g pitted black olives, finely chopped
1 garlic clove, crushed
4 anchovy fillets, finely chopped
1 tbsp capers, drained and finely chopped
1 tbsp red wine vinegar
1 bunch of basil, leaves torn
sea salt and freshly ground black pepper
extra-virgin olive oil

METHOD:

Preheat the oven to 210°C/190° fan/Gas mark 7.

Heat the wine in a small pan over a medium heat until hot but not bubbling. Add the couscous and saffron, stir, turn off the heat and set aside until all of the wine is absorbed.

Using a fork, fluff up the couscous and lay out on a plate. Coat the chicken breasts in the flour, then the egg and then the couscous, pressing it evenly over the chicken until fully coated.

Place the chicken on a wire rack above a baking tray and cook in the centre of the oven for 20–25 minutes or until fully cooked.

Meanwhile, prepare the puttanesca. In a large bowl combine the tomatoes, olives, garlic, chopped anchovy fillets, capers, red wine vinegar, torn basil and a good pinch of salt and pepper. Drizzle well with extra-virgin olive oil and stir well.

To serve, spoon the puttanesca onto a plate and top with the couscous crusted chicken. Scatter some extra basil leaves over the top and give it a good drizzle of extra-virgin olive oil.

BAKED COD WITH PROSCIUTTO AND RUSTIC PEA AND MINT MASH

Quick to cook and ridiculously easy, this dish is one of my classics, especially when there's little time to rustle up something healthy and tasty. The key is a good thick piece of cod, good-quality prosciutto and lots of lemon, salt and pepper to serve it with.

INGREDIENTS:

4 cod loin fillets
4 slices prosciutto
500g Maris Piper potatoes, peeled and cut into large chunks
250g frozen garden peas
50g butter
25ml double cream
1 sprig of mint, very finely chopped
sea salt and freshly ground black pepper

TO SERVE:

4 lemon wedges

METHOD:

Preheat the oven to 200°C/180°C fan/Gas mark 6.

Line a baking sheet with baking parchment. Season the cod loins with salt and pepper and place on the tray. Top each cod loin with a prosciutto slice and cook in the oven for 15 minutes.

Bring a large pan of salted water to the boil and boil the potatoes for 10 minutes. Add the peas and continue to cook for further 5 minutes until the potatoes are soft. Drain, then add the butter and double cream and mash using a potato masher. Add the finely chopped mint and stir well.

Remove the cod loins from the oven and serve with the pea and mint mash and a lemon wedge on the side.

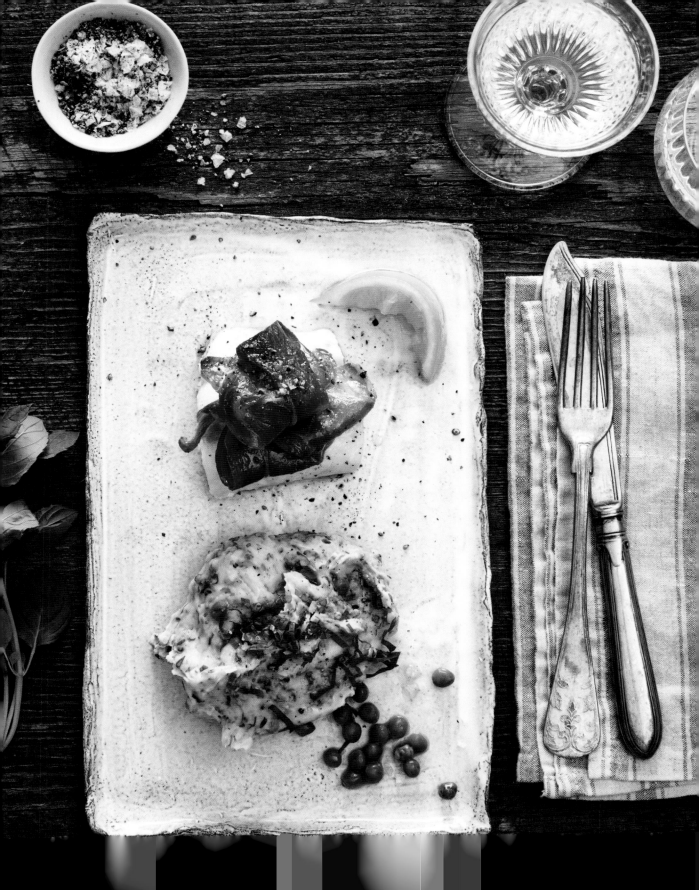

PRAWN, CHORIZO AND BEETROOT BARLEY RISOTTO

Pearl barley is one of my store cupboard staples, I love it; its texture and nuttiness is so satisfying, and it doesn't need constant stirring or attention. You can prepare everything and walk away, leaving it to cook. Not only does this dish look enticing but the salty sweet flavours from the chorizo and beetroot make it a comforting dish. You'll want seconds!

SERVES
4

INGREDIENTS:

olive oil
1 onion, finely chopped
1 garlic clove, finely chopped
300g pearl barley
100ml red wine
1 litre good-quality chicken stock
2 cooked beetroots, diced
200g cooking chorizo, diced
200g raw king prawns
50g feta
a handful of rocket leaves

METHOD:

Heat the olive oil in a heavy-based pan over a medium heat and fry the onion for a few minutes until soft. Add the garlic and continue to cook for a further two minutes.

Add the pearl barley to the pan, stirring until all the grains are coated in the oil. Add the red wine and allow it to bubble.

Add the chicken stock and beetroot to the pan and season with salt and pepper. Stir well, cover and cook for 20–25 minutes on a medium-low heat.

Place a small pan over a medium heat and fry the diced chorizo until crispy. Remove from the pan and drain on kitchen paper. Add the prawns to the pan to cook in the chorizo oil until pink and cooked through.

Check the pearl barley: if not all of the liquid has reduced, whack up the heat until it's bubbled away.

Remove from the heat and stir through the chorizo and prawns.

To serve, scatter with crumbled feta, fresh rocket and a drizzle of the chorizo cooking oil.

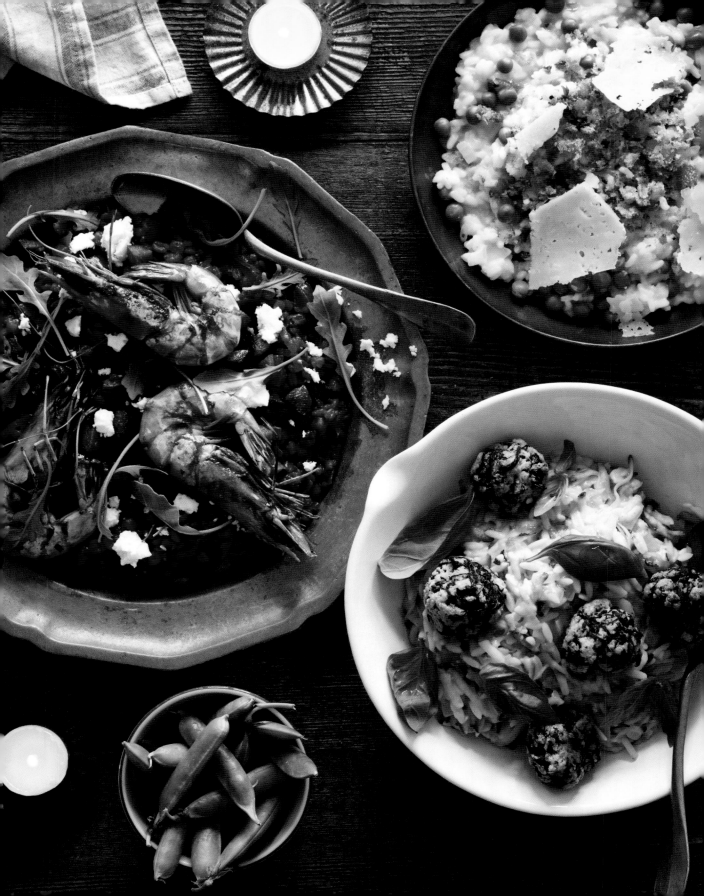

COURGETTE AND CHICKPEA BURGERS
WITH WHIPPED FETA AND PICKLED CUCUMBER

SERVES
4

Veggie burgers are delicious. A friend of mine decided to become a vegetarian recently, and the lack of burger choices was a problem. Wanting to help, I made this courgette and chickpea burger for her. It was a resounding success.

INGREDIENTS:

1 large courgette, grated
1 x 400g tin chickpeas, drained
1 red onion, finely chopped
3 heaped tbsp plain flour
a large handful of grated
Cheddar cheese
2 eggs, beaten
1 tsp chilli flakes
200g feta at room temperature
80g cream cheese at room
temperature
1 cucumber
1 tbsp malt vinegar
2 tsp salt
1 tsp sugar
olive oil, for frying

TO SERVE:

2 seeded burger buns
lettuce

METHOD:

Pop the grated courgette into a clean tea towel, season with salt and bring the corners of the towel together, wringing out as much liquid as you can.

In a large bowl combine the courgette, chickpeas, red onion, 1 tablespoon flour, and Cheddar cheese. Mash well using a potato masher or a fork until you have a combined mixture. Add the eggs and chilli flakes and mash again.

Divide the mixture into four and shape into patties. Coat with the remaining flour and pop in the fridge for 30 minutes to firm up.

Meanwhile, make the whipped feta. Crumble the feta and add to a food processor along with the cream cheese. Pulse for a couple of minutes until smooth and creamy.

To make the pickled cucumber, shave the cucumber into ribbons and place in a bowl with the vinegar, salt and sugar. Set aside for a few minutes.

Heat a glug of olive oil in a pan over a medium heat and cook the burgers for a few minutes on either side until golden brown and cooked through.

To assemble the burgers, place some lettuce on the bottom bun, then top with the burger, whipped feta and pickled cucumber.

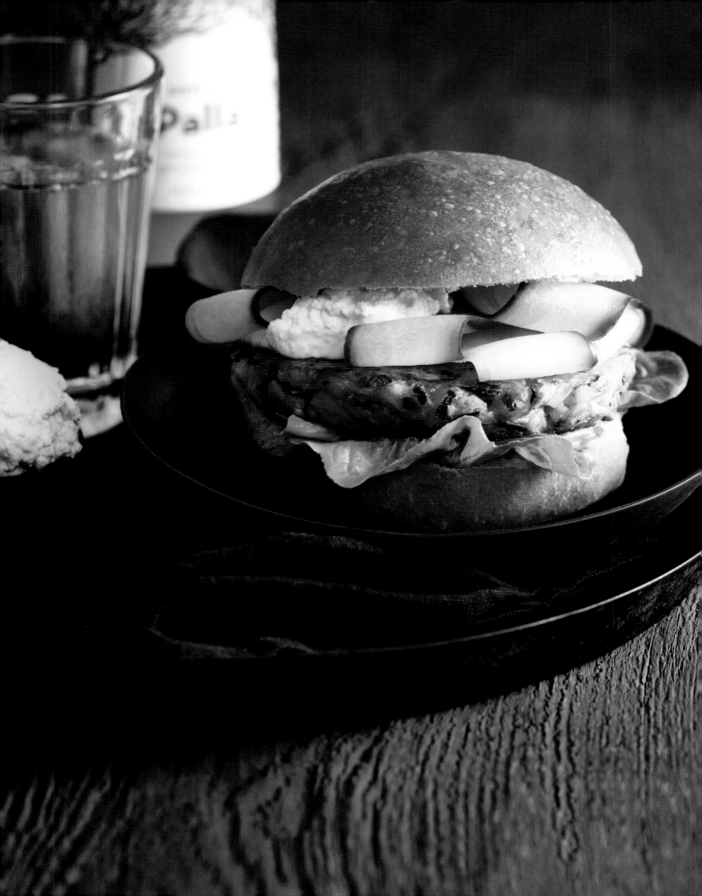

AMERICAN-STYLE BANQUET

My ultimate food indulgence is American voodoo wings, shrimps, as many sticky BBQ ribs as I can muster, lashings of blue cheese dip and endless frozen margaritas. This would be my last meal, all washed down with an intolerable amount of hot sauce.

A good number of our friends are guys, and it's the best type of raucous fun having a big crowd of them round to watch the game while the girlfriends catch up over a glass or two. Then we all dive into a feast of beers, sticky ribs and chocolate peanut butter cake. The sausage balls, mac and cheese, brownie cake and pork ribs can all be prepared in advance, then stuck in the oven as soon as everyone arrives.

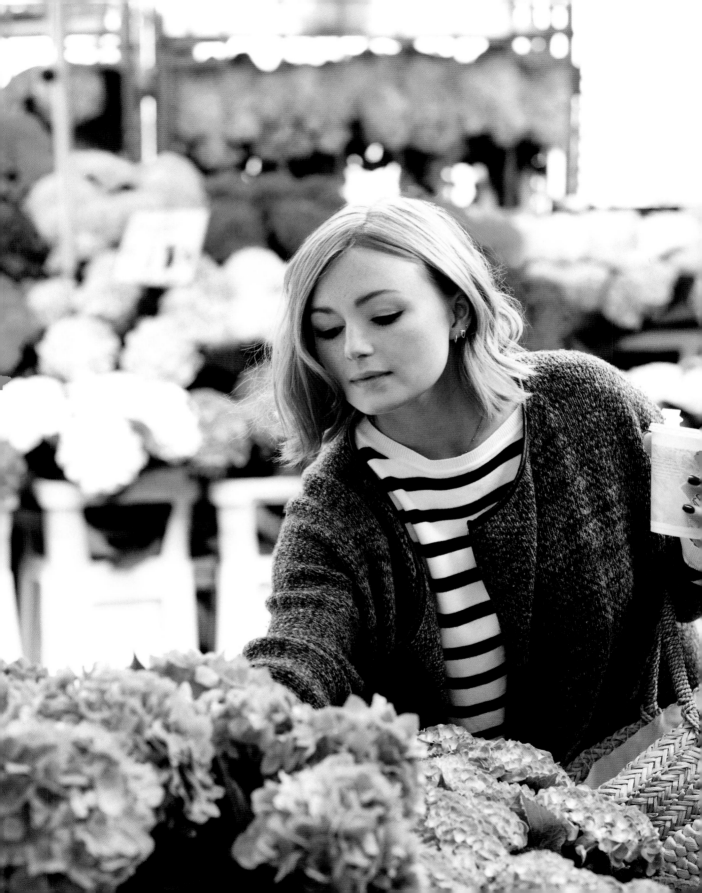

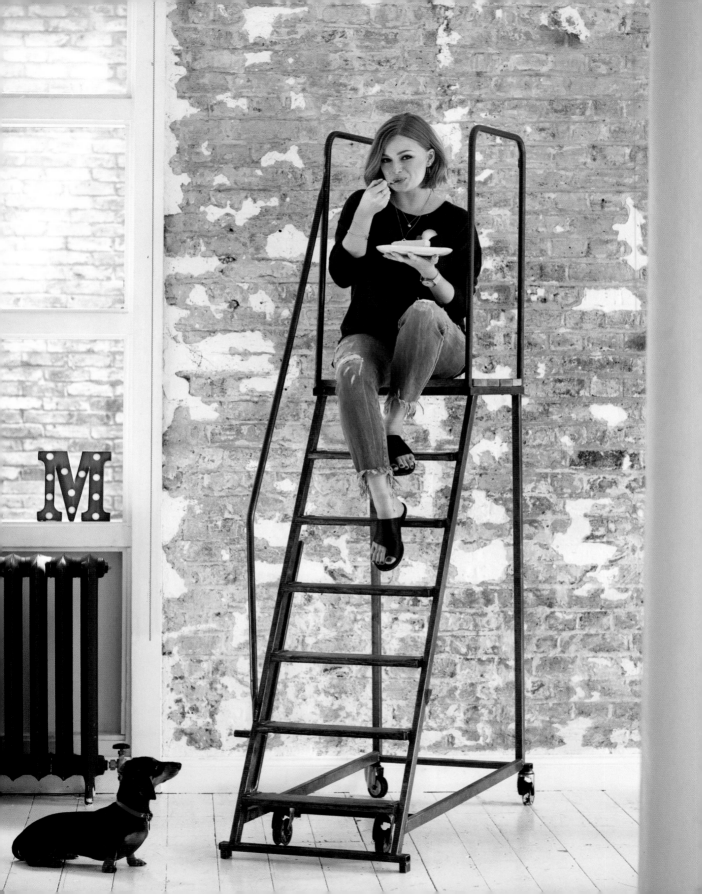

PUDDINGS AND SWEET TREATS

"Life is uncertain. Eat dessert first."
Ernestine Ulmer

PUDDINGS AND SWEET TREATS

My love for sweet things doesn't match my love for savoury foods. Sometimes, however, I crave the gooiest, sweetest and most decadent puddings or cakes. When this happens, these are my go-to recipes.

Death By Chocolate and Peanut Butter Brownie Cake (p 159) is exactly what it says on the tin: a decadent cake-brownie that silences the room every time. My grandfather's favourite, Lemon and Raspberry Vicky Sponge (p 162), is perfect for afternoon tea. Raspberry and Rose Jelly Cheesecake (p 154) and Nan's Lemon Mousse with Toasted Coconut (p 177) are both light, so perfect for the summer.

Much to my Swedish photographer's dismay, there are also Pimm's, Cointreau and Raspberry Jellies (p 167) in here because, like many Brits, I simply love a bit of sneaky booze in my pud.

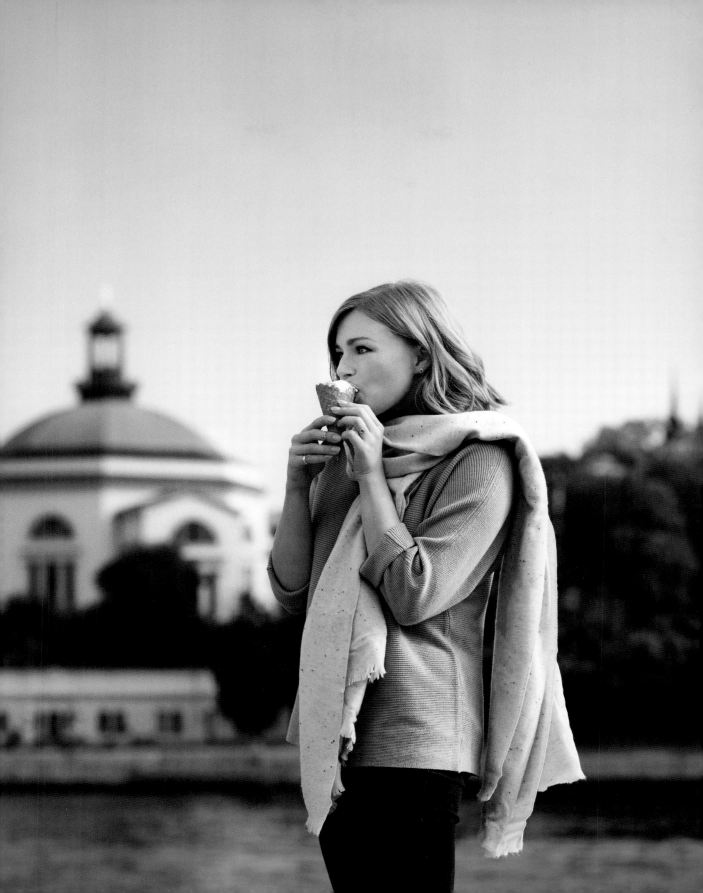

RASPBERRY AND ROSE JELLY CHEESECAKE

SERVES
8 – 12

I first made this cheesecake for my family when I was a teenager. It started off as a lime jelly cheesecake, then slowly progressed into first a chocolate orange cheesecake and finally the more refined raspberry and rose jelly cheesecake. This is a cheesecake like no other. If you're looking for a classic American, thick paste of a cheesecake, then I'm afraid this isn't that. But trust me, it's something much, much better.

INGREDIENTS:

butter, for greasing
250g plain digestive biscuits, crushed
100g unsalted butter, melted
1 x 135g pack Hartley's raspberry jelly cut into chunks
½ x 410g can evaporated milk
200g soft cream cheese
2 tsp rose essence
a handful of fresh raspberries and a few clean rose petals to decorate

METHOD:

Heavily grease the base and sides of a 20cm spring form tin.

In a bowl, mix together the crushed biscuits and the melted butter and press evenly into the bottom of the tin. Pop in the fridge to set.

Dissolve the jelly in 100ml boiling water and set aside.

In another bowl, whisk the evaporated milk until thickened and then whisk in the soft cheese until thick and creamy.

Add the rose essence to the jelly mixture and then fold into the whisked evaporated milk and cheese. Pour over the digestive base and refrigerate for at least 2 hours until firm.

To decorate, place some rose petals around the rim of the cake and top with an upside-down raspberry.

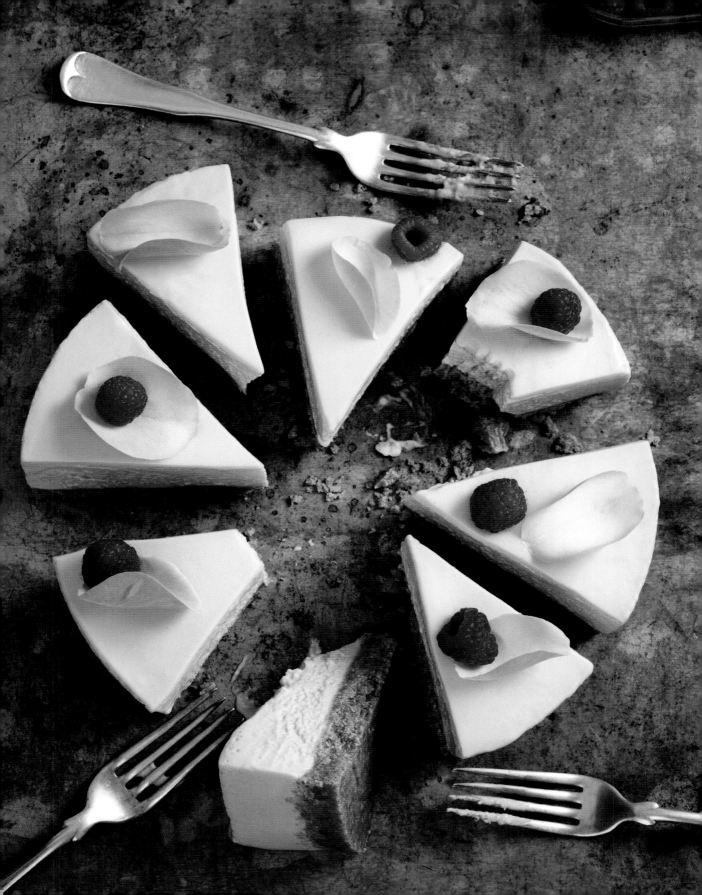

PEACH AND THYME FILO TARTE TATIN

SERVES
4

I don't think I have ever met anyone who didn't like a tarte Tatin. I would die for it, but a soggy pastry base can ruin the whole experience. Thinking of this, I tested a filo base; I suspected it would be an excellent substitute to the traditional puff pastry because it's much crispier, and as it turns out, it works very well. This peach and thyme tart is decadent, but dare I say, a little lighter due to the filo. So, you can get away with having more than one slice!

INGREDIENTS:

85g unsalted butter, cubed
120g caster sugar
2 sprigs of thyme
2 ripe peaches, cut into segments
6 sheets filo pastry
2 tbsp unsalted butter, melted

METHOD:

Preheat the oven to 200°C/180°C fan/Gas mark 6.

Place a 20cm ovenproof frying pan over a medium heat and melt the cubed butter and sugar over a medium heat, without stirring, until it becomes a caramel.

Lay the sprigs of thyme down in the caramel and top with the peach slices. Cook for a couple of minutes until softened, then remove from the heat.

Lay down a sheet of filo onto the work surface, brush with some melted butter and lay another sheet on top. Repeat this process with all 6 sheets and then lay the pastry over the top of the pan, carefully tucking the pastry in at the edges to create a snug lid. Brush with a little melted butter and pop into the oven for 15–20 minutes or until golden brown.

To serve, carefully place a plate on top of the pan and in, one swift movement, turn it upside-down.

Serve the tarte tatin whole for everyone to dig in with some good-quality vanilla ice cream on the side.

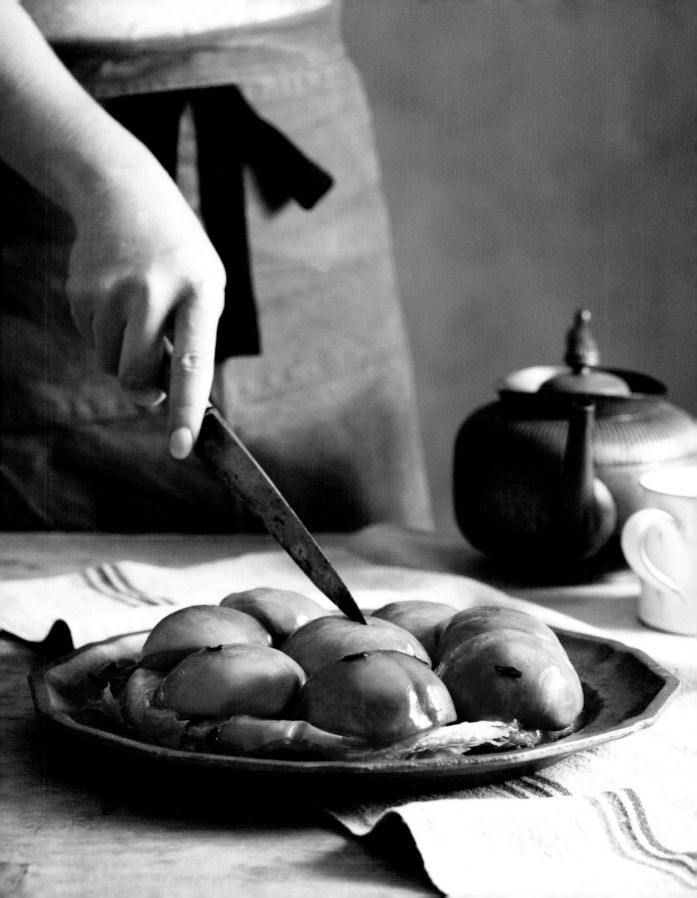

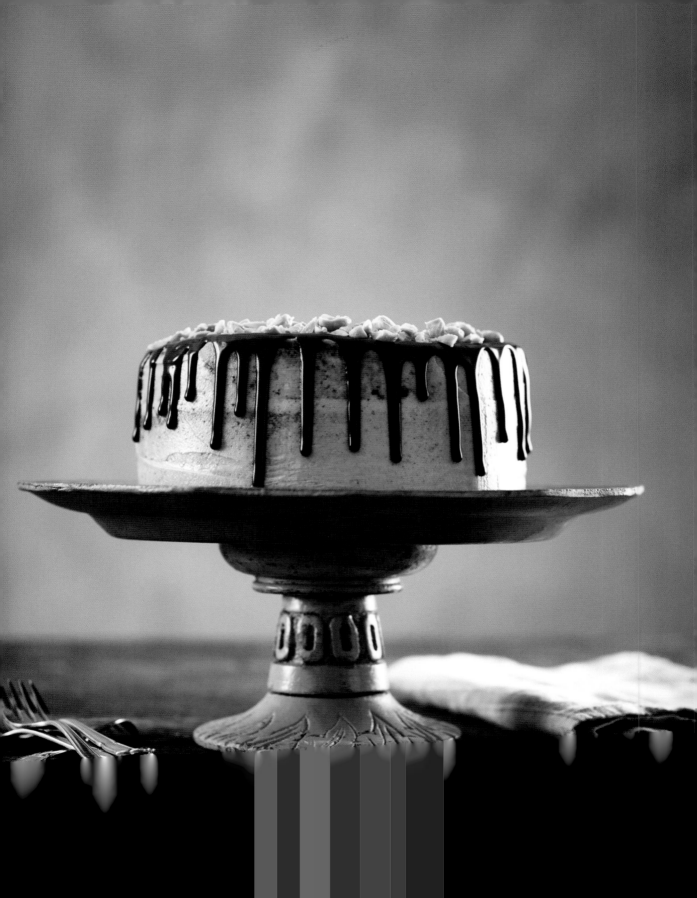

DEATH BY CHOCOLATE AND PEANUT BUTTER BROWNIE CAKE

SERVES
8 – 12

Chocolate and peanut butter, a delicious combination now merged into a cake, brownie-style. A sponge that's denser than your average cake makes this become something a bit more sinful. And I'm not ashamed to admit it was originally a mistake. I wanted a fluffy sponge, but I rather liked this misdemeanour and so embraced it. Enjoy!

INGREDIENTS:

350g unsalted butter at room temperature, plus extra for greasing

350g self-raising flour, plus more for dusting

150g good-quality dark chocolate, broken-up into pieces

150g good-quality milk chocolate, broken-up into pieces

350g caster sugar

6 eggs, beaten

2 tsp baking powder

8 tbsp good-quality cocoa powder

1 tbsp vanilla paste or extract

METHOD:

Preheat the oven to 180°C/160°C fan/Gas mark 4.

Grease three 20cm round cake tins with butter and then dust with flour until they're fully coated. Cut 3 strips of greaseproof paper and line each tin with a strip going across the middle. This helps lift the sponges from the tins once cooked.

Make a bain-marie by placing a non-metallic bowl over a pan of boiling water, making sure the base of the bowl isn't touching the base of the pan. In the bowl, melt the dark and milk chocolate. Once the chocolate is fully melted, remove the bowl from the simmering water and allow to cool.

In a separate bowl, beat the butter with the sugar for 10 minutes until soft, or for 5 minutes if you have an electric whisk. Slowly mix in the beaten eggs and then gently fold in the sifted flour, baking powder, cocoa powder and vanilla paste with a metal spoon, scraping the mixture up from the bottom to the top in circular motions until the mixture is just about combined. If the mixture feels stiff, add some milk to loosen it a little. At this point, gently fold in the melted chocolate.

continued overleaf

DEATH BY CHOCOLATE AND PEANUT BUTTER BROWNIE CAKE
CONT...

INGREDIENTS:

FOR THE ICING:

200g unsalted butter at
room temperature
400g good-quality smooth
peanut butter
400g icing sugar
80g soured cream at room
temperature
sea salt

TO DECORATE:

100g good quality dark
chocolate, broken up into
pieces
25g unsalted peanuts

EQUIPMENT:

3 x 20cm sandwich tins and an
electric whisk (the whisk isn't
essential but makes the job
easier)

METHOD CONTINUED:

Divide the mixture evenly between the 3 tins and bake in the middle of the oven for 25–30 minutes until the cakes have risen and are springy to the touch. Allow to cool for about 10 minutes in the tins, then using the greaseproof paper strips, gently lift up and transfer to a wire rack to cool completely.

To make the peanut butter icing, beat the butter, peanut butter and icing sugar until smooth. Add in the soured cream and a good pinch of salt and continue to beat for another minute.

When the cakes have fully cooled, halve the icing and then divide one of the halves in half again. Place one of the cake layers onto a cake stand and spread evenly with one quarter of icing. Top with another cake layer, and spread on the other quarter of the icing. Add the final cake layer and spread the remaining icing over the top and sides of the cake, using a palette knife to smooth. You want the icing to lightly cover the cake, but the sponge to show through.

To decorate, slowly melt the chocolate over a bain marie over a medium heat. Once fully melted, drizzle the edge of the cake with the chocolate and allow it to drip down the sides. Sprinkle the crushed peanuts around the edge and allow to set fully before serving.

FROZEN CHOCOLATE BANANA LOLLIES

SERVES
4

No prize for originality on this one, but if you're after a sweet treat and don't want the ice cream drawer, this is a great alternative. Kids love them, too. Mix and match your toppings: nuts, seeds and dried fruit all work well. Be creative!

INGREDIENTS:

4 bananas
a mixture of milk, dark or white chocolate, broken into pieces
a mixture of hazelnuts, almonds or any other nuts, toasted
a mixture of dried fruits such as cranberries and banana chips, coconut or orange rind

METHOD:

Trim the ends of each banana and stick a wooden ice cream stick into one end.

Place the bananas on some greaseproof paper and freeze for at least 2 hours, preferably overnight.

Once the bananas are frozen, melt as much chocolate as you fancy over a bain-marie and dip in the bananas until fully coated. Scatter with the nuts and/or dried fruit and pop back in the freezer for 10 minutes to firm up before serving.

LEMON AND RASPBERRY VICKY SPONGE

SERVES
8 – 10

The Great British Victoria sponge is everyone's favourite. My version has a couple of twists. Lots of lemon zest lifts the sponge, and the soured cream takes off the sweet edge. Try orange zest, or adjusting the amount of soured cream to your taste. My Grandad is a huge fan – and if it's good enough for him at over 100 years old, it's good enough for everyone.

INGREDIENTS:

115g soft unsalted butter, plus extra for greasing
115g self-raising flour, plus extra for dusting
115g caster sugar
2 eggs, beaten
1 tsp vanilla paste or extract
zest of 1 unwaxed lemon

FOR THE BUTTERCREAM:

100g unsalted butter
3 tsp soured cream
150g icing sugar, plus extra for dusting
2 heaped tbsp good-quality raspberry jam
fresh strawberries, to decorate

EQUIPMENT:

2 x 20cm sandwich tins and an electric whisk (the whisk isn't essential but makes the job easier)

METHOD:

Preheat the oven to 180°C/160°C fan/Gas mark 4.

Grease the cake tins with butter and then dust with flour until they're fully coated. Cut 2 strips of greaseproof paper and line each tin with a strip going across the middle. This helps when you come to lift the sponges from the tins once cooked.

Pop the butter into a bowl and, using an electric whisk, beat the butter on the slowest setting until it turns pale in colour. Add the caster sugar and whisk until light, soft and creamy. Gradually add the eggs and continue to beat, then add the vanilla paste and half the lemon zest. Once fully combined, sift in the four and use a metal spoon to gently fold it in until incorporated and you have a thick batter.

Divide the cake mixture between the two tins and bake in the centre of the oven for 20–25 minutes until golden brown and the sponge is springy to the touch.

Allow the cakes to sit in their tins for 5 minutes before turning out onto a wire rack. Allow to cool completely.

Meanwhile, make the buttercream. Whisk together the butter, soured cream and icing sugar until smooth.

Stir the jam to loosen and add the remaining lemon zest. Spread onto one half of the cake. Spread the buttercream over the other half and sandwich the two together. Dust with icing sugar, decorate with the strawberries and serve!

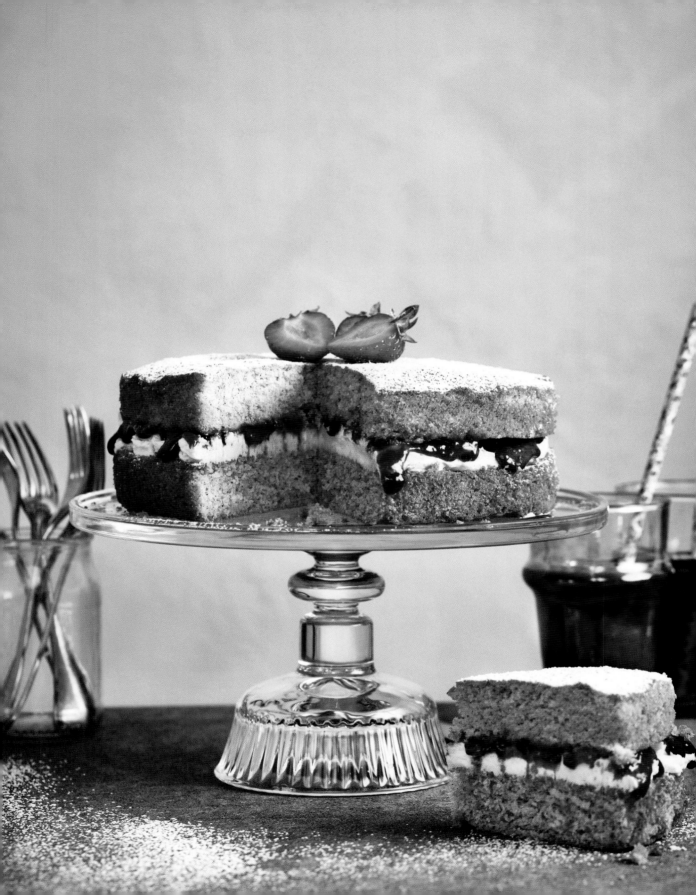

PORTUGUESE ALMOND CAKE

SERVES
8 – 12

Spending a lot of time in Portugal as a kid and teenager meant I got to taste a wide variety of Portuguese pastries and cakes, and trust me, some of them were incredible. The best has to be their almond cake, stuffed with lots of ground almonds and almond essence, which makes it very flavoursome but moist too. I like to top mine with even more almond icing – too much is never enough.

INGREDIENTS:

100g unsalted butter, plus extra for greasing
100g self-raising flour, sifted, plus extra for dusting
200g caster sugar
3 eggs, beaten
100g ground almonds
1 tsp almond essence
1 tbsp brandy

FOR THE BUTTERCREAM:

100g unsalted butter
3 tsp soured cream
1 tsp vanilla paste
1 tsp almond essence
150g icing sugar
flaked almonds, toasted, to decorate

EQUIPMENT:

1 x 20cm sandwich tin and an electric whisk (the whisk isn't essential but makes the job easier)

METHOD:

Preheat the oven to 180°C/160°C fan/Gas mark 4.

Grease the cake tin with butter and then dust with flour until it's fully coated. Cut 1 strip of greaseproof paper and line the tin with the strip going across the middle. This helps lift the sponge from the tin once cooked.

Using an electric whisk, cream together the butter and sugar until light and fluffy. Gradually add the eggs, beating well with each addition. Fold in the flour and ground almonds and add the almond essence and the brandy.

Pour the mixture into the prepared cake tin and bake in the oven for 45 minutes or until a skewer comes out clean.

Allow the cake to sit in its tin for 5 minutes before turning out onto a wire rack. Allow to cool completely.

To make the icing, beat together the butter, soured cream, vanilla paste, almond essence and icing sugar until smooth.

Use a spatula to spread the icing over the top of the cooled cake and decorate with flaked almonds.

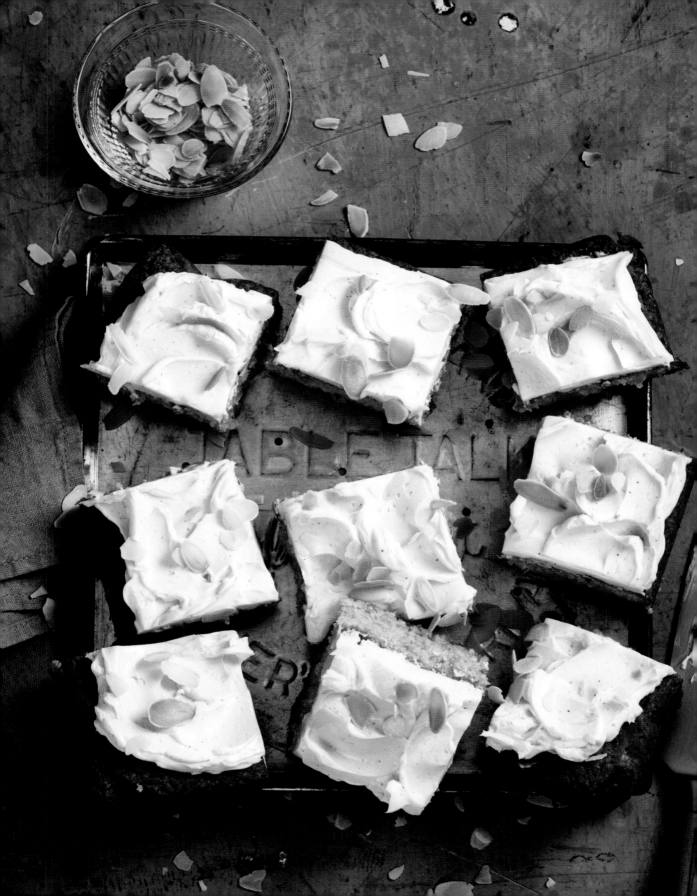

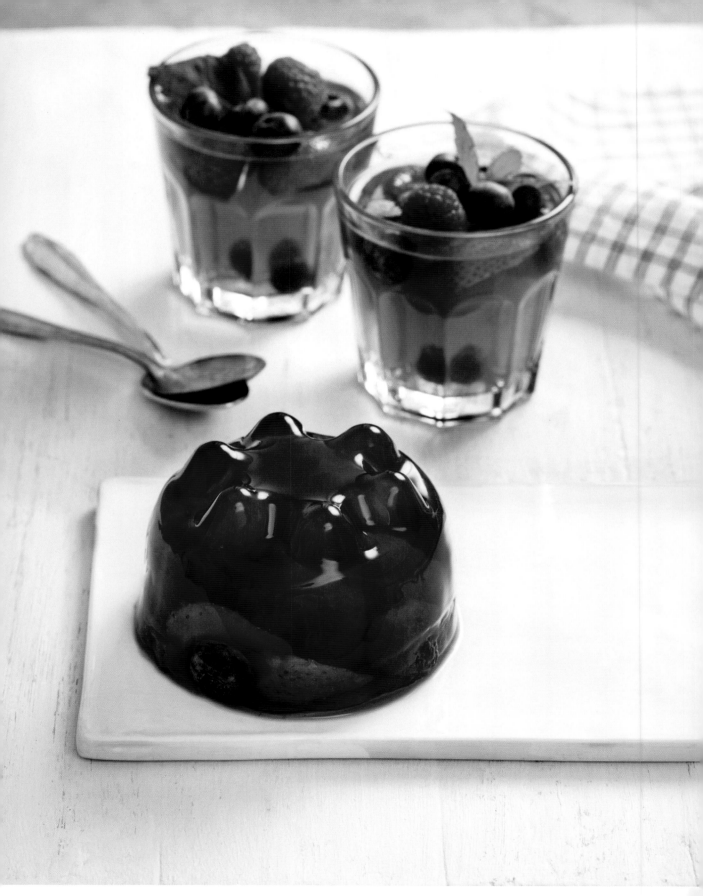

PIMM'S, COINTREAU AND RASPBERRY JELLIES

SERVES
4

My food photographer for this book – Susanna – made me laugh when shooting this recipe. She said, "Jelly is so retro. Nobody likes jelly anymore." Well, she doesn't know us Brits well enough then, because we LOVE the stuff! What's more, we love an alcoholic jelly. Whip this out on a hot day and you'll be mega popular, I promise you that.

INGREDIENTS:

6 gelatine leaves
300ml lemonade
150ml ginger beer
150ml Pimm's
1 tbsp Cointreau
a selection of raspberries, blueberries and strawberries, cut in half and into segments
fresh mint and extra berries to garnish

METHOD:

Soak the gelatine leaves in cold water for a few minutes.

Place a pan over a low-medium heat, pour in the lemonade, ginger beer, Pimm's and Cointreau liqueurs and gently heat, but don't allow it to simmer.

Turn off the heat, squeeze all of the liquid from the gelatine and add to the pan. Stir gently until all the gelatine has dissolved.

Divide the fruit between glasses or jelly moulds and carefully pour over the jelly mixture. Put the jellies in the fridge and leave to set overnight.

When you're ready to serve, half fill a bowl with hot water and dip the glasses or moulds in the water for about 5 seconds to help release the jelly from their moulds. Give them a bit of a wiggle, turn out onto a plate and garnish with fresh mint and extra berries.

ROSE-SHAPED APPLE TARTS WITH WALNUT CRUST

SERVES
4

These tarts are pretty and work perfectly for pudding, teatime, or even a fancy breakfast. The crust is made from walnuts, too, so if you're catering for someone who follows a gluten-free diet this is perfect for them.

INGREDIENTS:

200g walnut halves

50g unsalted butter, melted

1 egg white

1 tbsp caster sugar

8 tbsp Greek yoghurt

1 tsp vanilla paste or extract

4 Pink Lady apples

juice of 1 lemon

honey

sea salt

EQUIPMENT:

2 x 10cm loose-bottomed tart tins. (You can buy these super cheaply online.)

METHOD:

Preheat the oven to 190°C/170°C fan/Gas mark 5.

In a mini blender, blend the walnuts until you have fine crumbs. Tip into a bowl and mix with the melted butter, egg white, caster sugar and a pinch of salt. Press the mixture evenly into tart tins and bake in the oven for 8–10 minutes. Turn off the oven and keep the door ajar, leaving them in the oven to cool completely.

Mix together the Greek yoghurt and vanilla paste and spoon into the cooled cases.

Prepare the apples by slicing them in half, removing the core with a teaspoon and thinly slicing into half moon-shaped segments. Pop them into a bowl with the lemon juice and 300ml water, then microwave on high for 2 minutes. Set aside to cool completely.

To make the roses, create a line of apple segments with their straight edges facing you, overlapping the apple segments from left to right, creating a caterpillar of apple slices. Very carefully, roll the segments up, from left to right, until you form a rose shape.

Using a little honey, stick the edge of the outermost apple segment onto the base of the apple rose to hold it in place, then carefully lay on top of the vanilla Greek yoghurt.

Drizzle the roses with honey and serve immediately.

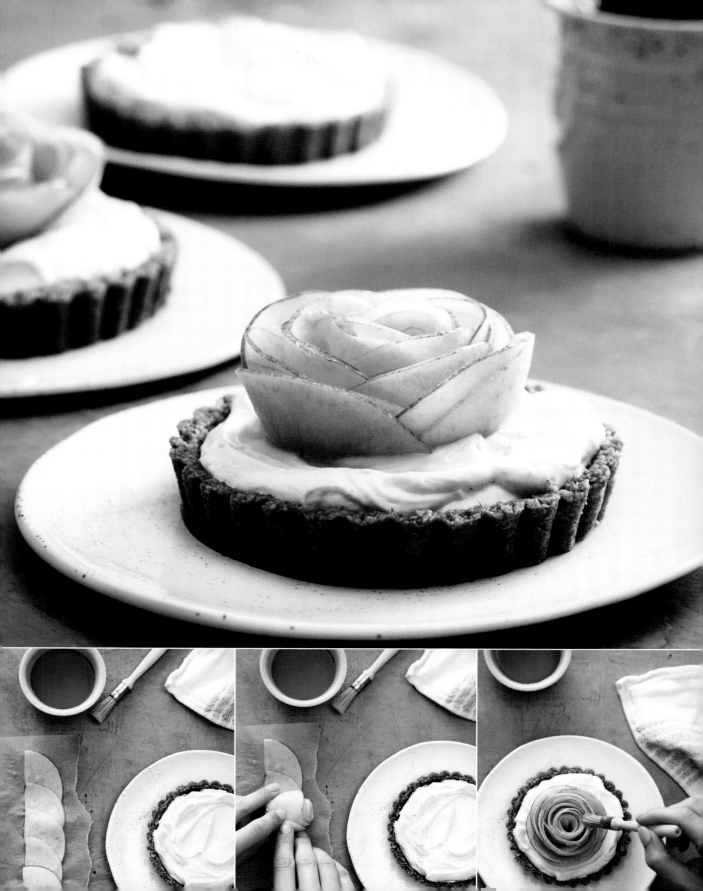

BISCOTTI, HONEY-BAKED FIGS AND CHEESE

Crunchy biscotti, stinky cheese and honey-baked figs, washed down with a glass of sweet wine. A delicious, simple-to-put-together, heavenly plate.

INGREDIENTS:

FOR THE BISCOTTI:

285g plain flour

150g caster sugar

1 tsp baking powder

¼ tsp sea salt

3 eggs

1 tsp vanilla extract

1 tsp almond extract

FOR THE HONEY-BAKED FIGS:

12 fresh figs, cut in half

1 tbsp honey

TO SERVE:

Saint Vernier, or another strong cheese

METHOD:

Preheat the oven to 180°C/160°C fan/Gas mark 4.

First make the biscotti. In a bowl mix together the flour, caster sugar, baking powder and salt. In a separate bowl mix together the eggs, vanilla and almond extracts and then slowly add to the dry ingredients. Beat well until it comes together to form a sticky dough.

Divide the dough in 2 and roll into 2 fat sausages, squashing them down a little. Bake in the oven for 20–25 minutes, then remove from the oven and allow to cool.

Meanwhile, place the figs on a baking tray, cut-side up, and drizzle with honey.

Once the biscotti are cool enough to handle, slice into pieces about 2cm thick. Lay them on their side and place among the figs and bake in the oven for 15–20 minutes. Turn the biscotti halfway through cooking.

Once the biscotti are cooked and the figs are nice and sticky, remove from the oven and allow to cool completely. Serve with a potent cheese such as Saint Vernier and a crisp dessert wine.

NO-FUSS CHOCOLATE PIZZA

We've all been there: those days when you can't be bothered to cook, or you've forgotten family or friends are on their way for lunch. Crisis! So you rustle up some pasta or pop some sausages in the oven. This recipe is unashamedly a process of layering shop-bought ingredients to create something a little bit different, which will indulge the sweet tooth of every chocolate-lover out there. Minimal effort, zero stress. Result.

INGREDIENTS:

2 tortilla wraps
4 tbsp chocolate spread
2 tbsp crushed toasted hazelnuts
12 raspberries
1 tsp icing sugar

TIP:

Try my Homemade Chocolate Spread on page 210

METHOD:

Preheat the oven to 220°C/ 200°C fan/ Gas mark 7.

Spread the chocolate spread on one side of each wrap. Scatter with the hazelnuts, pop onto a wire rack over a baking tray and bake for 8–10 minutes until the edges start to crisp up.

Remove from the oven, drop over the fresh raspberries and dust with icing sugar.

Cut into four slices and serve immediately.

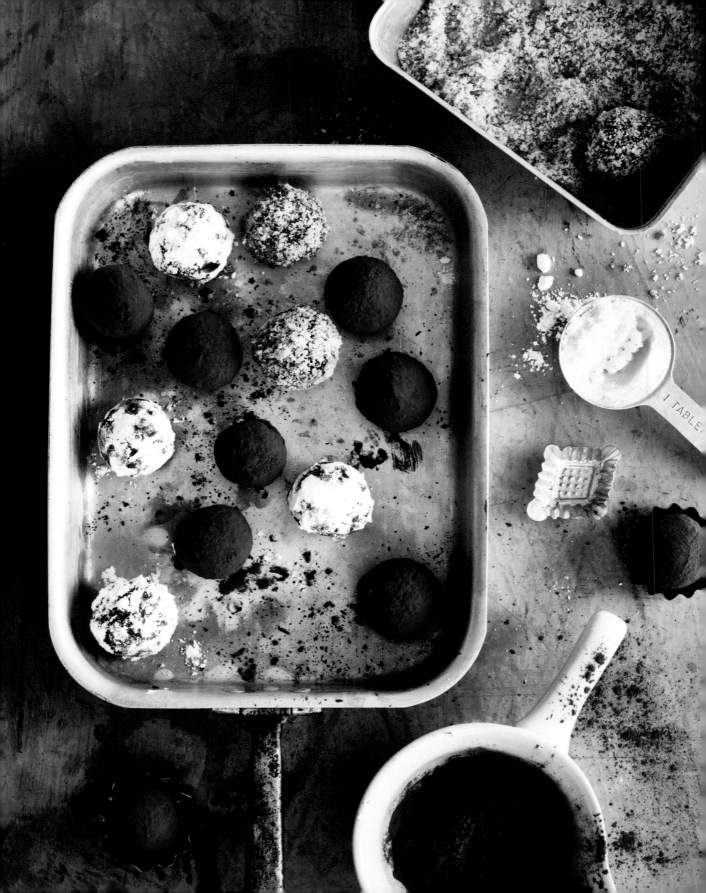

AMARETTO CHOCOLATE TRUFFLES

MAKES
OVER A DOZEN

For a lovely homemade gift or a special occasion I love to make chocolate truffles. Embarrassingly easy, incredibly impressive, these little bites are always a hit.

Feel free to add your alcohol of choice. Rum, crème de menthe and coffee liquor work equally well.

INGREDIENTS:

150g good-quality dark chocolate, finely chopped
150ml double cream
25g unsalted butter
2 tbsp Amaretto liqueur
1 tbsp Greek yoghurt
cocoa powder for dusting
icing sugar, for dusting
crushed hazelnuts, for dusting

METHOD:

Place a bowl in the fridge to chill.

Make a bain-marie by placing a non-metallic bowl over a pan of boiling water, making sure the base of the bowl isn't touching the base of the pan. In the bowl, melt the dark chocolate.

Add the double cream, butter and Amaretto liqueur and gently combine with the chocolate and remove from the heat.

Stir in the Greek yoghurt and transfer to the chilled bowl and set aside to cool completely.

Once cooled, cover with clingfilm and put in the fridge overnight until fully set.

To create the truffles, use a teaspoon or a melon baller to scoop balls of the chocolate mixture. Roll in your hands and then roll in cocoa powder, icing sugar or the crushed hazelnuts. Transfer to a plate and repeat with the remaining chocolate mixture. Keep these in the fridge and they'll keep for a couple of weeks… if they last that long!

CINNAMON AND CHAI TEA POACHED PEARS

SERVES
4

This smells divine: chai reminds me of my teenage years. I hadn't yet acquired the taste for coffee, and when I wanted a hot drink, a chai latte was my choice. It's wonderfully fragrant and sweet, second helpings are often required. Serve with ice cream or a dollop of cream.

INGREDIENTS:

2 chai tea bags
150g caster sugar
1 cinnamon stick
4 pears, ripened but not too soft

METHOD:

Select a saucepan that can fit all four pears on their sides snuggly without crushing them when the lid is on.

Pour 300ml boiling water into the empty pan and add the chai tea bags, sugar and cinnamon stick. Bring to the boil for 10 minutes to dissolve the sugar, then squeeze out the teabags and discard along with the cinnamon stick.

Peel and core the pears and cut off the bottoms so they can stand up.

Place the pears in the pan on their sides and bring to a simmer, pop the lid on and poach for 15–20 minutes, depending on how ripe your pears are. Turn the pears half way through cooking to get a nice even colour.

Once the pears are soft, remove from the pan and set aside. Bring the poaching liquid back up to the boil and reduce for about 10 minutes until you have a syrup.

Serve the pears standing up with the syrup poured over.

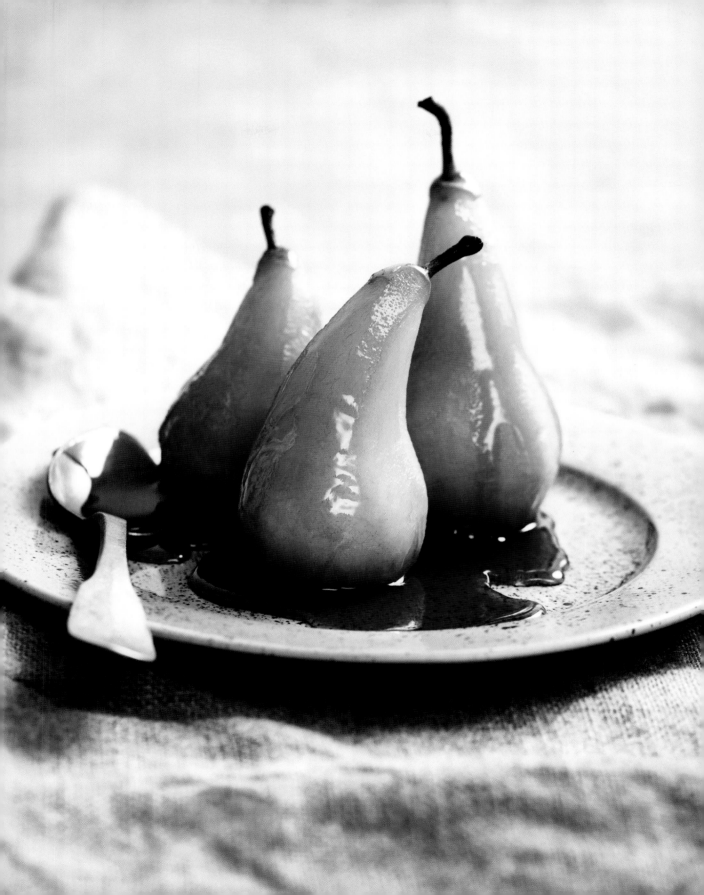

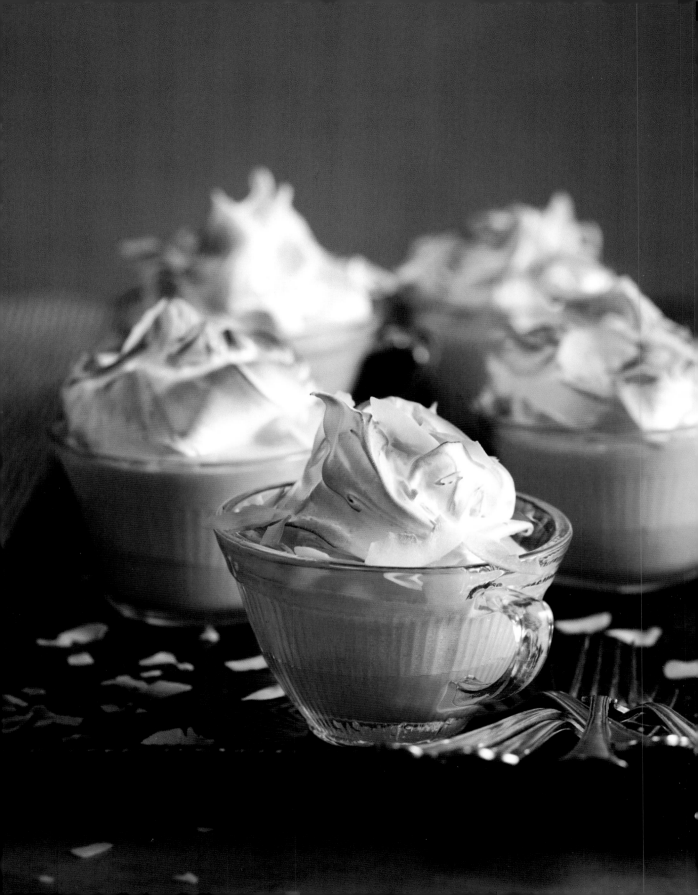

NAN'S LEMON MOUSSE WITH TOASTED COCONUT

SERVES
4

My Nan's lemon mousse is something I will always remember fondly. This uses my Lemon, Lime and Thyme Curd (p 210) at the bottom and Italian meringue for the top. It's a show stopper pudding – elegant, not too over-the-top and a conversation piece.

INGREDIENTS:

FOR THE MOUSSE:

zest of 3 unwaxed lemons, with a little set aside for decoration
60ml lemon juice
180g golden caster sugar
4 eggs, separated
155g unsalted butter, cubed
4 tbsp lemon curd

FOR THE ITALIAN MERINGUE:

120g granulated sugar
2 egg whites
4 tbsp toasted coconut flakes

EQUIPMENT:

a kitchen thermometer would be usful here

METHOD:

Place most of the lemon zest, the lemon juice, sugar and egg yolks
in a bain-marie over simmering water and stir constantly for 10 minutes, or until the mixture coats the back of a metal spoon. Gently whisk in the butter, a cube at a time. Remove from the heat and allow to cool.

In a very clean bowl, whisk the egg whites until stiff peaks are formed.

Using a metal spoon, fold half of the egg whites into the lemon mixture and then very gently fold in the remaining egg whites.

Spoon 1 tablespoon of lemon curd into the bottom of 4 serving glasses and then top with the lemon mousse. Pop in the fridge for at least 2 hours to set.

To make the Italian meringue, put the sugar and 50ml water in a small pan and dissolve over a medium heat.

Meanwhile, in another clean bowl, whisk the egg whites until they form peaks. Set aside.

Turn up the heat on the sugar and water and bring to the boil until it reaches 120°C. Once at temperature, slowly pour the sugar mixture into the egg whites and beat continually, until you end up with really glossy, stiff egg whites.

To serve, spoon 1 tablespoon of the Italian meringue on top of the set mousse and either pop under a hot grill for a few minutes until browned or caramelise with a kitchen blowtorch. Scatter with the toasted coconut flakes and serve.

MOJITO FROZEN YOGHURT

MAKES
2 litres

As a kid I used to pop a carton of yoghurt in the freezer as a snack. This version I make from scratch with a nod to the mojito. Leave out the rum if you're making for children.

INGREDIENTS:

500g natural yoghurt
100g caster sugar
zest of 2 limes
juice of 1 lime
1 tbsp rum
1 tbsp chopped mint leaves

METHOD:

In a bowl, mix together all the ingredients and pop into a zip-up sandwich bag. Freeze for 4 hours. Every hour or so, give the bag a bit of a squish to keep it moving.

If you over-freeze the yoghurt or want to make ahead, don't worry: just allow to thaw a little and give it a good squish before serving. You want a frozen but still loose consistency.

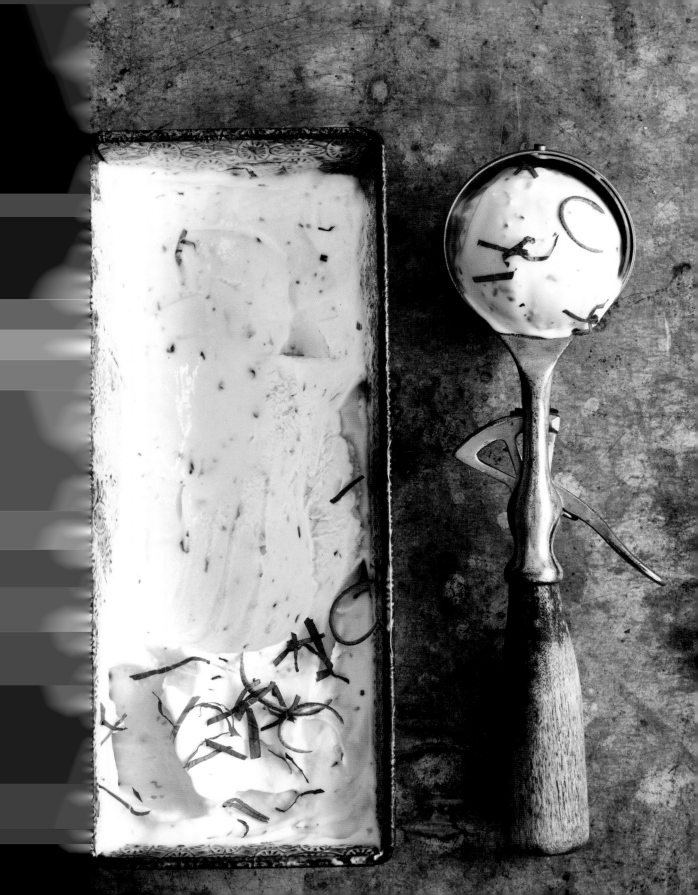

LAVENDER AND HONEY CUPCAKES

MAKES
12

As a little girl, I often made cupcakes with my mum. Today making them is rather nostalgic and something I really enjoy. These are more grown-up with a subtle lavender flavour coming through. You can buy dried lavender online or in the baking section in some supermarkets.

INGREDIENTS:

40g unsalted butter at room temperature
120g plain flour
140g caster sugar
1½ tsp baking powder
120ml milk
1 egg
1 tsp lavender essence

FOR THE ICING:

80g unsalted butter at room temperature
160g icing sugar
1 tbsp honey
1 tsp lavender essence
purple food colouring
dried lavender to decorate, optional

EQUIPMENT:

12-hole cupcake or muffin tin lined with 12 paper cases

METHOD:

Preheat the oven to 170°C/150°C fan/Gas mark 3.

In a bowl, add the butter, flour, caster sugar and baking powder and use an electric whisk to beat until all the butter is incorporated and you have a sand-like texture.

In a separate bowl, mix together the milk, egg and lavender essence and slowly add to the dry mixture, mixing until you have a batter.

Pour the batter into the cupcake cases, about a heaped tablespoon in each, and bake in the centre of the oven for 15 minutes or until lightly golden and springy to the touch. Remove from the oven and allow to rest for 5 minutes and then turn out onto a wire rack to cool completely.

To make the icing, whisk together the butter, icing sugar, honey and lavender essence together for a couple of minutes until smooth. Add as much purple food colouring as you like, then put in the fridge for 15–20 minutes or until firm.

Ice the cupcakes using the back of a spoon and garnish with a dried sprig of lavender.

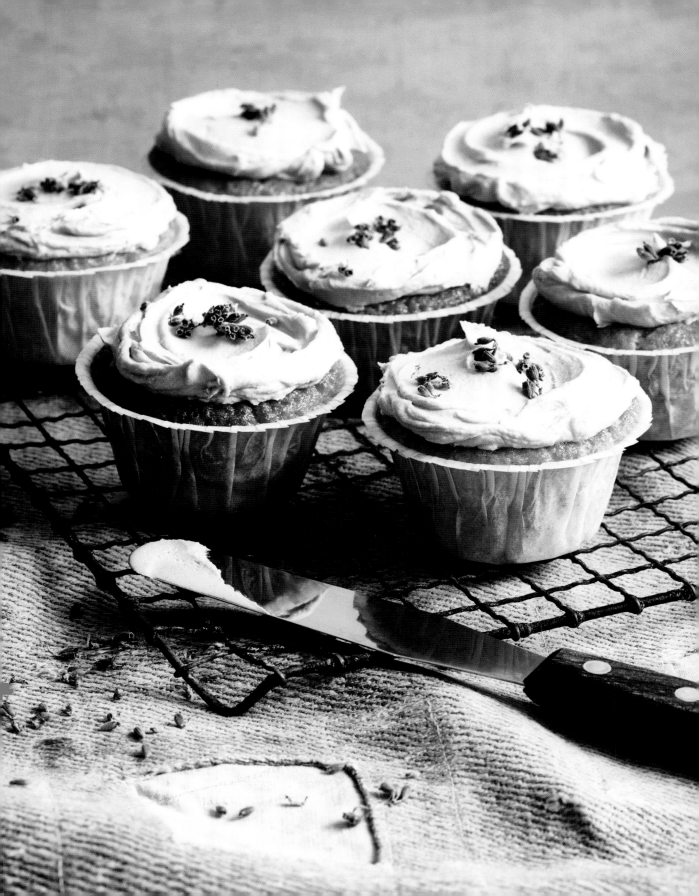

OREO CUPCAKES

MAKES
12

What's there to say? Oreos in a cupcake. Heavenly. Loved by young and old.

INGREDIENTS:

40g unsalted butter
100g plain flour
20g good-quality cocoa powder
140g caster sugar
1½ tsp baking powder
120ml milk
1 egg
1 tsp vanilla paste
18 Oreo biscuits

FOR THE ICING:

160g unsalted butter
360g icing sugar
8 Oreo biscuits, crushed into fine crumbs

EQUIPMENT:

12-hole cupcake or muffin tin lined with 12 paper cases

METHOD:

Preheat the oven to 170°C/150°C fan/Gas mark 3.

In a bowl, add the butter, flour, cocoa powder, caster sugar and baking powder and use an electric whisk to beat until all the butter is incorporated and you have a sand-like texture.

In a separate bowl, mix together the milk, egg and vanilla paste and slowly add to the dry mixture, mixing until you have a batter.

Put 1 whole Oreo in the bottom of each paper case and add a heaped tablespoon of the cupcake batter. Bake in the centre of the oven for 15–20 minutes or until springy to the touch.

Remove from the oven and allow to rest for 5 minutes and then turn out onto a wire rack to cool completely.

To make the icing, whisk together the butter and icing sugar for a couple of minutes until smooth and then stir in the crushed Oreos. Put in the fridge to set until firm.

Ice the cupcakes and cut the remaining 6 Oreos in half. Stand half an Oreo in the icing on top of each cupcake.

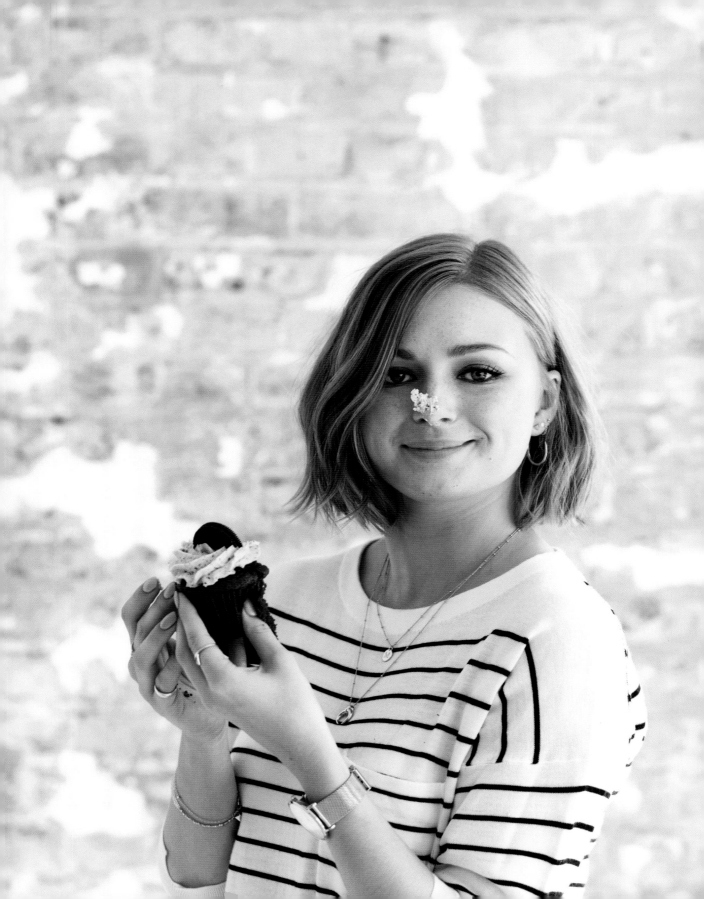

There's nothing quite as special as a proper English afternoon tea. Start with Prosecco and the obligatory smoked salmon and cucumber sandwiches, then follow with this selection of sweet treats. My Vicky Sponge is a twist on the classic, and what afternoon tea would be complete without Pimms? Or, more specifically my Pimms, Cointreau and Raspberry Jellies? Then soothing cups of English tea to follow, coupled with my easy "Cherry Bakewell" Bites.

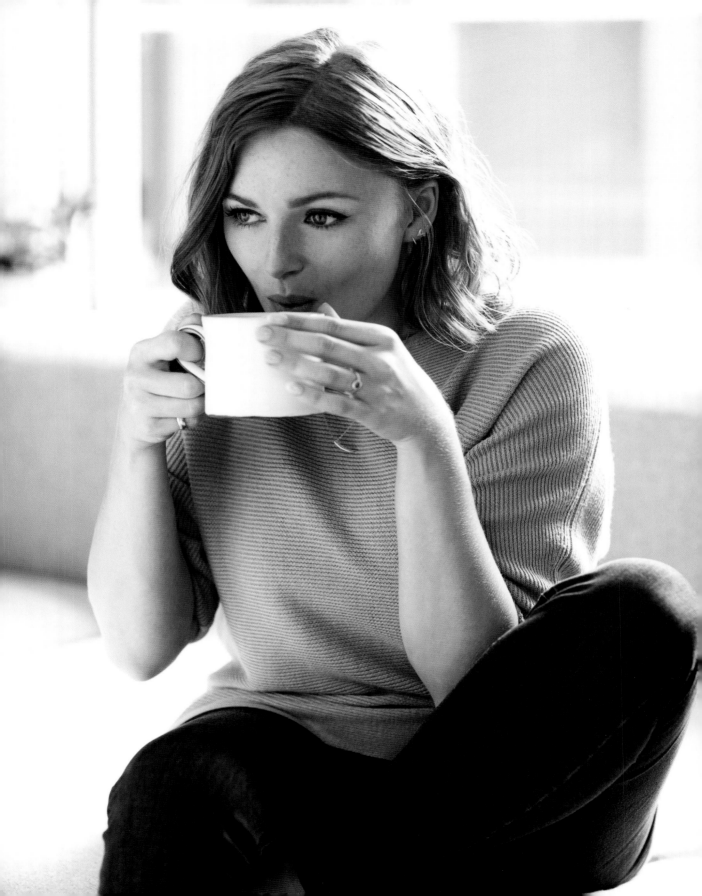

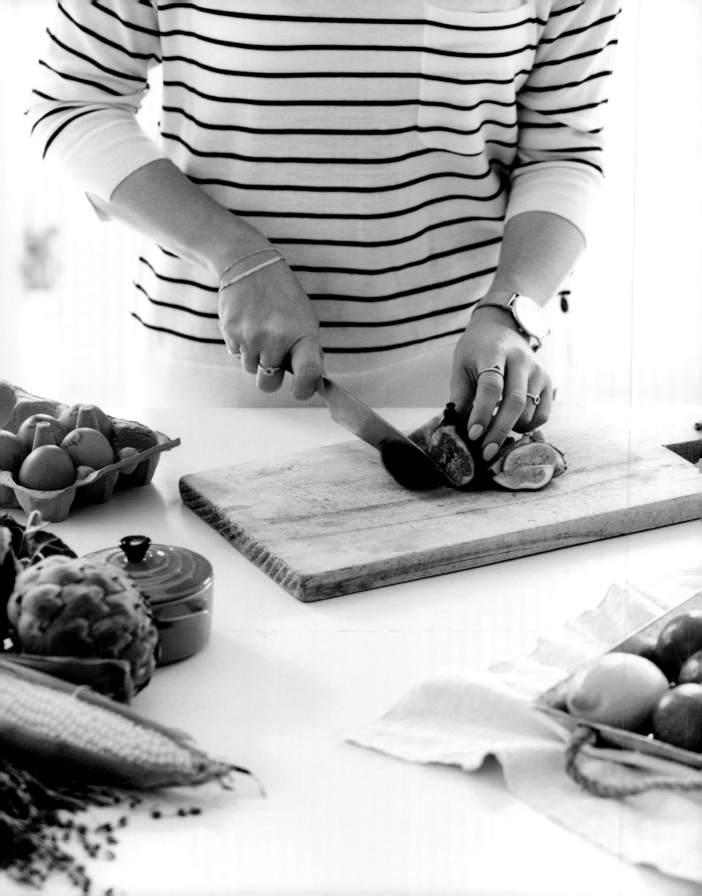

SIDES, SNACKS AND SAUCES

"A balanced diet is a cookie in each hand."
Unknown

SIDES, SNACKS AND SAUCES

This is the home of the dishes that you wouldn't necessarily eat all by themselves (although the sides are good enough to have on their own as a light dinner), but they are crucial if you want to get the most out of meal, or have a craving for something to nibble at. These are the unsung heroes of cooking, the wingmen of your main dish, or brilliant gap-fillers for when you want to veg out on the sofa but avoid going the whole hog with a family-sized grab bag of crisps.

Side dishes such as Honeyed Dijon Green Beans with Toasted Almonds (p 200), Shredded Sprout and Pomegranate Salad (p 198) and Rose Petal Rosemary and Garlic Potatoes (p 196) bring a bit of oomph to your dinner when you want to impress.

For the times when you need a snack that isn't processed, I have Buffalo Roasted Chickpeas (p 202), Chai Spice and Sea Salt Popcorn (p 207) and Cherry Bakewell Bites (p 197). Perhaps too good to share!

Finally, there are recipes for sauces, pestos, dips and spreads that can all be used alongside other dishes. If you make a jar, there's plenty of ideas and ways for using them throughout the book.

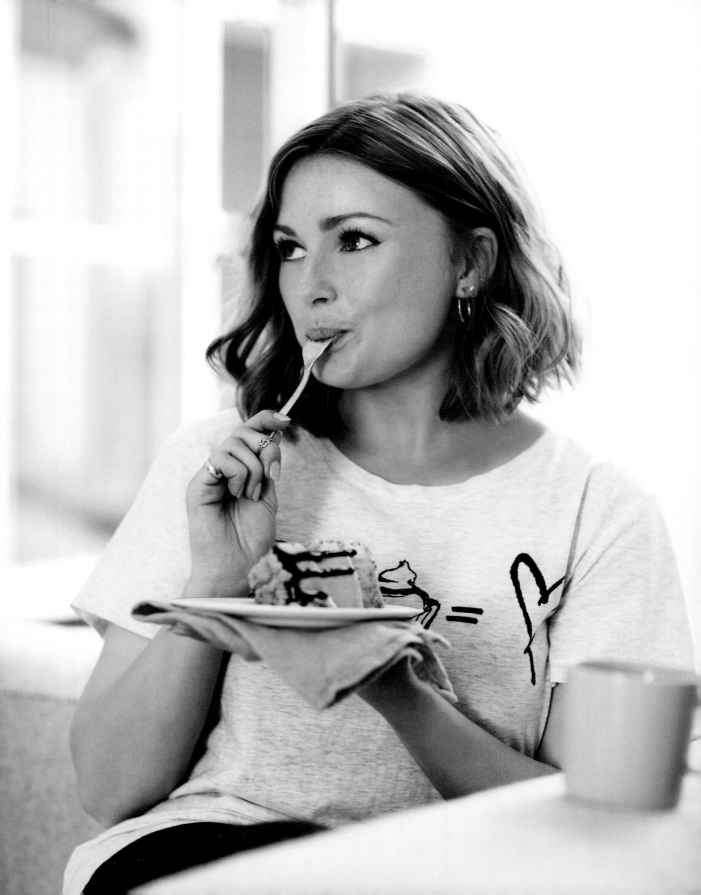

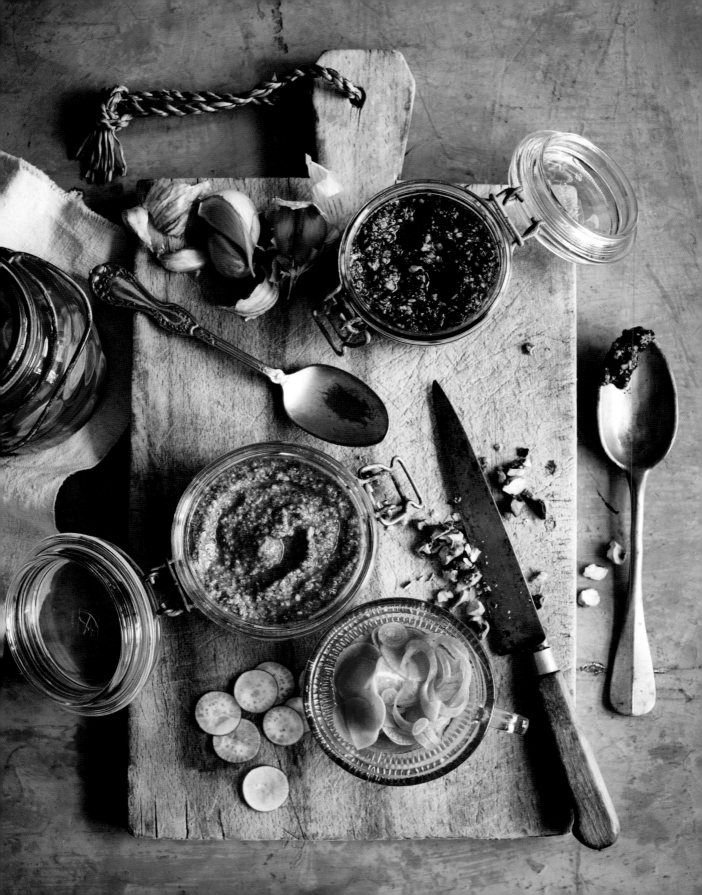

KALE AND PISTACHIO PESTO

MAKES
1 jar

INGREDIENTS:

4 large leaves of cavolo nero or
black kale
1 tbsp unsalted, shelled
pistachios
a handful of freshly grated
Parmesan cheese
½ garlic clove
100ml rapeseed or olive oil
juice of ½ lemon
sea salt

METHOD:

Blend together the first 4 ingredients, adding the oil slowly as
you blend until you get a runny consistency.
   Add the lemon juice and blend until smooth.
Season with salt.
   The pesto will keep for up to 1 month in the fridge.

DILL AND WALNUT PESTO

MAKES
1 jar

INGREDIENTS:

1 bunch of fresh dill, finely
chopped
1 bunch of fresh basil, finely
chopped
2 tbsp walnuts, finely chopped
a handful of freshly grated
Parmesan cheese
½ garlic clove
100ml olive oil
juice of ½ lemon
sea salt

METHOD:

Blend together the first 5 ingredients, adding the oil slowly as
you blend until you get a runny consistency.
   Add the lemon juice and blend until smooth. Season with
salt.
   The pesto will keep for up to 1 month in the fridge.

HOMEMADE BUTTER 3 WAYS

Making your own butter is so satisfying and very easy. Feel free to be creative and try lots of different ingredients! These are my favourite flavours, perfect for slathering over a roast chicken or adding to steamed vegetables. The cinnamon and orange sugar is perfect on crumpets or French toast.

SUNDRIED TOMATO AND PARMESAN BUTTER

INGREDIENTS:

1 litre double cream
2 tbsp finely chopped sundried tomatoes
4 tbsp freshly grated Parmesan cheese
1 tsp sea salt

DILL, LEMON AND PARSLEY BUTTER

INGREDIENTS:

1 litre double cream
1 tbsp lemon zest
2 tbsp finely chopped fresh dill
2 tbsp chopped flat-leaf parsley
1 tbsp sea salt

CINNAMON-SUGAR AND ORANGE RIND BUTTER

INGREDIENTS:

1 litre double cream
2 tbsp granulated sugar
1 tsp cinnamon
1 tbsp orange rind

METHOD:

Whip the double cream in a food processor and on a medium speed until thick. Continue to mix past the point of thick cream, and the cream will start to collapse and thicken, separating into butter and buttermilk.

Once you've got this consistency, fold out onto a cold and very clean sieve over a bowl and allow to drain well.

Pour away the buttermilk and mix the butter with your hands or a fork to get any further excess buttermilk out of the butter.

Knead it well and then add any flavours you fancy.

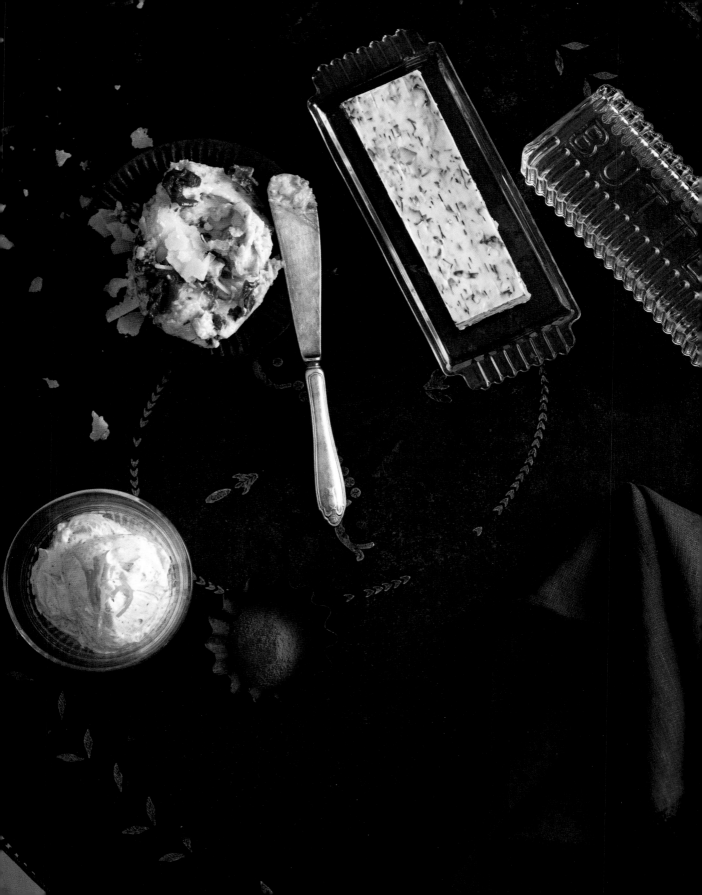

TANGY PEANUT DIP

This goes well with Rainbow Salad Rolls (p 64) and Bang Bang Chicken Salad (p 78) but also works nicely as a dipping sauce for crudités, or served over brown rice, fish or chicken.

MAKES
1 jar

INGREDIENTS:

2 heaped tbsp crunchy peanut butter
1 tbsp toasted sesame oil
3 tbsp light soy sauce
1 tbsp fish sauce
1 tbsp honey
juice of 1 lime
1 tsp chilli flakes

METHOD:

Mix together all the ingredients until combined. The lemon might curdle the peanut butter; if that happens, just add a drop more sesame oil and mix until smooth.

The dip will keep for up to 1 week in the fridge.

SWEET CHILLI JAM

Delicious with Fried Chicken Thighs (p110), cheese or cold meats.

MAKES
1 jar

INGREDIENTS:

8 red peppers, deseeded and roughly chopped
8 red chillies, roughly chopped
1 red onion, roughly chopped
4 garlic cloves, peeled
50g ginger, peeled roughly chopped
1 x 400g tin cherry tomatoes
750g caster sugar
250ml red wine vinegar
1 tbsp sea salt

METHOD:

To make the jam, tip the peppers, chillies, red onion, garlic and ginger into a food processor and blitz until very finely chopped.

Spoon into a heavy-based pan with the cherry tomatoes, caster sugar, red wine vinegar and salt. Bring everything to the boil, skimming off any frothy scum that floats up to the surface, so you end up with a clear jam. Reduce the heat to a simmer and cook for about 50 minutes, stirring occasionally.

Once the jam is ready, pour into a sterilised jar and allow to cool. It will keep for up to 1 month in the fridge.

RADISH AND RED ONION PICKLE

The perfect topping for pulled pork sandwiches, hamburgers and tacos.

MAKES
1 litre

INGREDIENTS:

200ml red wine vinegar
200ml apple cider vinegar
3 tbsp caster sugar
1 tbsp sea salt
1 medium red onion
15–20 radishes

METHOD:

Pour the vinegars, sugar, salt and 200ml water into a saucepan and stir over a medium heat until the sugar and salt have completely dissolved.

Using a mandolin, slice the red onion and radishes – or, if you don't have one, slice very finely using a knife. Layer the red onion and radishes into sterilised jars and then pour the vinegar into the jars all the way to the top.

Tap the jars on a surface to bring any air bubbles to the top, pop the lid on and refrigerate.

The pickle will keep for up to 1 month in the fridge.

ROSE PETAL ROSEMARY AND GARLIC POTATOES

Follow the same method as with the apples in the Rose-Shaped Apple Tarts with Walnut Crust (p 168), but replacing apple slices with potato slices. Pop into a cupcake tray, and you've got some outrageously pretty potatoes to serve up alongside your Sunday Roast.

MAKES
6

INGREDIENTS:

unsalted butter
3 large potatoes – I like using
Desirée potatoes
1 garlic clove, crushed
1 tsp dried rosemary
1 tbsp olive oil
sea salt and freshly ground
black pepper

EQUIPMENT:

12-hole cupcake tray

METHOD:

Preheat the oven to 200°C/180°C fan/Gas mark 6.

Grease the cupcake tray and set aside.

Using a mandolin, finely slice the potatoes into a large bowl – or, if you don't have one, slice very finely using a knife. Add the garlic, rosemary, salt and pepper and olive oil and use your hands to toss the lot together.

To make the roses, create 6 lines of potato slices, overlapping from left to right, creating a caterpillar of potato slices. Very carefully, roll the segments up, from left to right, until you have 6 roses. Place in the prepared non-stick cupcake tray.

Cook in the oven for 20–25 minutes until golden and crispy.

"CHERRY BAKEWELL" BITES

MAKES

8 – 12

For those moments when you want to raid the cookie jar and you need a little something, these are perfect – they're made from fruit and nuts, but taste like cherry Bakewell tarts.

INGREDIENTS:

170g pitted Medjool dates

150g plain cashews

40g glacé cherries

40g ground almonds and extra for rolling

1 tsp almond essence

METHOD:

In a food processor pulse the dates, cashews, cherries, ground almonds and almond essence until they come together in a ball to form a sticky, grainy texture.

Wet your hands and grab a small, bite-sized amount of the mix. Roll in your hands to form a ball, then roll in the ground almonds to fully coat. Repeat with all the mixture and then pop the bites in the fridge to set.

These will happily keep for up to 1 week in an airtight container.

SHREDDED SPROUT AND POMEGRANATE SALAD

SERVES
6 as a side

Brussels sprouts are not just for Christmas! A fantastic way to use up sprouts, this is a delicious, versatile dish all year round. If you have a mandolin slicer, use it to get very finely shredded sprouts; otherwise, slice as finely as you can. Because the salad is left for 10 minutes before serving, the dressing marinates and wilts the leaves, so although this salad is raw, it's refreshing, not chewy.

INGREDIENTS:

500g Brussels sprouts
seeds of 1 pomegranate
1 tbsp pomegranate molasses, or use honey if you can't get hold of any
3 tbsp red wine vinegar
5 tbsp olive oil
zest and juice of 1 unwaxed lemon
zest and juice of 1 unwaxed orange
sea salt and freshly ground black pepper

METHOD:

Using a food processor or a mandolin, shred the sprouts until they're very finely chopped and add them to a bowl.

Add most of the pomegranate seeds to the bowl along with the molasses, red wine vinegar, olive oil and lemon and orange zest and juices.

Season well with salt and pepper and mix well. Set aside for at least 10 minutes.

Scatter with the remaining pomegranate seeds before serving.

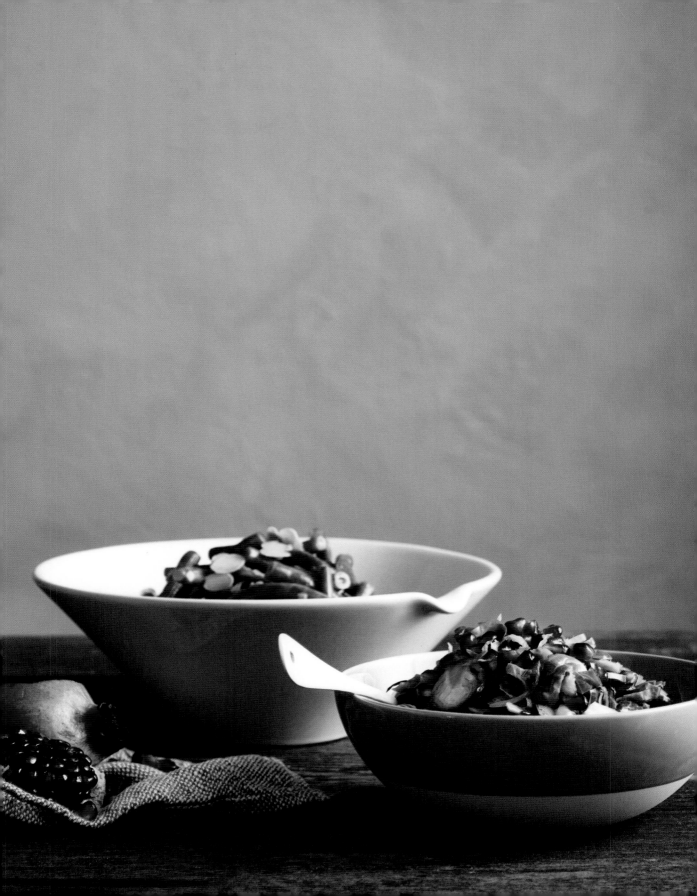

HONEYED DIJON GREEN BEANS WITH TOASTED ALMONDS

SERVES
6 as a side

A super simple but delicious side dish. This is the perfect accompaniment for a Sunday Roast or a juicy steak. Add a little more mustard if you prefer. Sweet, tangy and absolutely delicious, this also works as a cold dish for a buffet or picnic.

INGREDIENTS:

500g green beans
1 banana shallot, finely chopped
3 tbsp Dijon mustard
2 tbsp honey
1 tbsp red wine vinegar
1 tbsp olive oil
sea salt and freshly ground black pepper
2 tbsp flaked almonds, toasted

METHOD:

Place a large pan of salted water over a medium heat and bring to the boil.

Cook the green beans for 5–7 minutes, then drain and drop immediately into a bowl of iced water to stop the cooking process.

In a serving dish, add the finely chopped banana shallot, mustard, honey, red wine vinegar and olive oil and season well with salt and pepper.

Remove the beans from the ice water and drain onto kitchen paper, before adding to the bowl with the dressing. Toss well and top with the flaked almonds.

"CHOCOLATE BROWNIE" BITES

MAKES
8 – 12

If you really want an 11a.m. treat, this fruit and nut version tricks your brain into thinking you're eating a gooey brownie when you're loading up on some goodness. Keep these in an air-tight container in the fridge and they'll be fine for a couple of weeks.

INGREDIENTS:

170g pitted Medjool dates

150g cashews

40g walnut halves

1 tsp vanilla paste

2 tbsp good-quality cocoa powder

METHOD:

In a food processor pulse all of the ingredients, except the cocoa powder, until they come together in a ball to form a sticky, grainy texture.

Wet your hands and grab a small, bite-sized amount of the mix. Roll in your hands to form a ball, then roll into the cocoa powder. Repeat with all the mixture and then pop the bites in the fridge to set.

These will happily keep for up to 1 week in an airtight container.

SRIRACHA AND LIME BAKED CORN

This dish has a carefree street-food feel that makes it perfect for barbecues, warmer weather and al fresco eating.

SERVES
3

INGREDIENTS:

3 corn on the cobs, preferably with the husks still on
olive oil
100g butter
1 tsp of Sriracha (available at all Asian and major supermarkets)
zest of ½ lime
1 tsp sea salt

METHOD:

Preheat the oven to 200°C/180°C fan/Gas mark 6.

To prepare the corn, peel back the husks and tie with string. Coat in a little olive oil and bake in the centre of the oven for 30–35 minutes or until tender.

To make the butter, combine with the Sriracha, lime zest and salt and mix well. Transfer to a small serving bowl alongside the corn.

Serve the cobs with the butter spread over the hot kernals.

BUFFALO ROASTED CHICKPEAS

I love voodoo sauce on chicken wings, shrimp, you name it; I drink the stuff. These are a different take on crisps, nuts and wasabi peas. Simply bake a tin of chickpeas until crisp and cover in lashings of hot sauce. A tasty snack that's not deep fried.

SERVES
1 or 2 as a snack

INGREDIENTS:

1 x 400g tin chickpeas, drained
1 tbsp olive oil
sea salt and freshly ground black pepper
6 tbsp hot sauce, or as much as you can muster

METHOD:

Preheat the oven to 220°C/200°C fan/Gas mark 7.

In a bowl, mix together the chickpeas with the olive oil, salt and pepper and pour onto a baking tray. Spread them out evenly and bake in the oven for 25–30 minutes.

Remove the chickpeas from the oven and pour over half the hot sauce, then pop back in to oven for a few minutes. Repeat this process one more time, then allow to cool before serving.

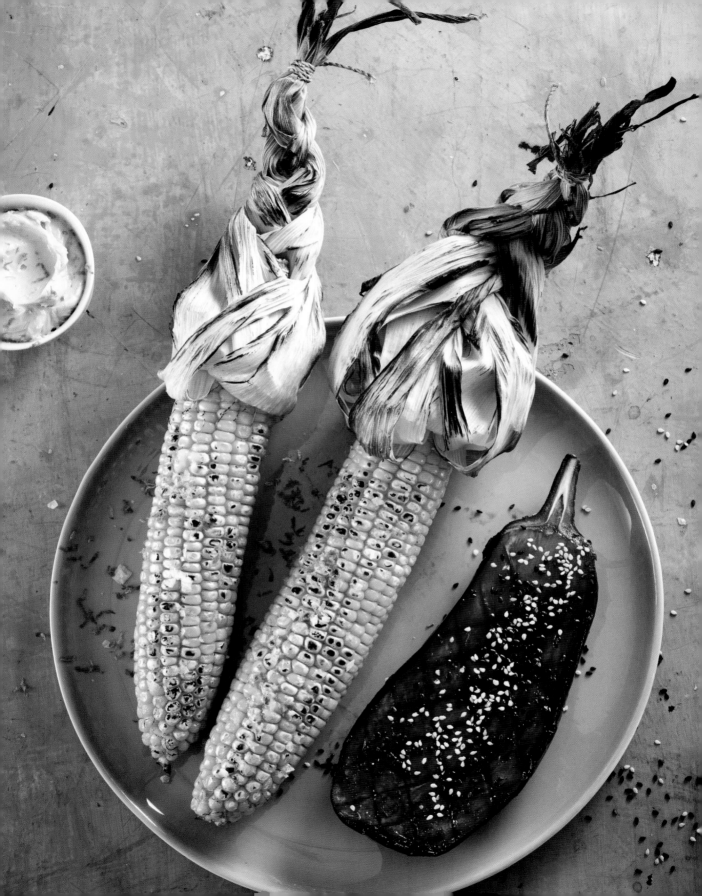

SWEET MISO-BAKED AUBERGINE

This is my ultimate Japanese dish. Nasu Dengaku is the name of the original, but this take on it has more easily available ingredients. Tender, succulent aubergine with a sweet, salty and tangy caramelised topping – absolutely delicious. Serve as a side or team with some greens and steamed rice to make it into a main dish.

INGREDIENTS:

2 x 18g sachets of miso paste (available at all larger supermarkets)
2 tbsp light soy sauce
1 tbsp soft brown sugar
1 tbsp toasted sesame oil
2 tbsp malt vinegar
1 tbsp vegetable oil
1 aubergine
1 tsp sesame seeds

METHOD:

Place a pan over a medium heat, then add the miso paste, soy, sugar, oil and vinegar and simmer for 8–10 minutes until sticky.

Preheat the grill to its highest setting.

Place a large pan over a medium–high heat and add the vegetable oil. Slice the aubergines in half, and score the flesh into criss-crosses. Once the oil is hot, fry the aubergine flesh-side down for 4–5 minutes until brown. Move from the pan to a baking tray and allow to cool skin-side down for a further 4–5 minutes.

Brush the aubergines with the miso sauce and place under the grill for 3–4 minutes until bubbling and caramelised.

Scatter with sesame seeds and serve immediately.

SHAVED APPLE AND FENNEL SALAD
WITH APPLE CIDER VINAIGRETTE

SERVES
4

I went to New York with my mother a few years ago and, as usual, we'd overindulged a bit too much the night before and went for a wander, stopping for a spot of lunch around the Rockefeller Center. I was craving something green and so ordered what was simply described as an "apple salad". Fitting, since we were in the Big Apple.

This is my take on it. A crisp and refreshing salad with fragrant fennel and a honey, mustard and apple cider vinegar dressing. This salad is so delicious I could eat it by itself, but it also works really well accompanying creamy dishes because the acidity cuts through the richness. Try teaming with my Ultimate Mac and Cheese (p 111) for a simple but delicious supper. If you can't find curly endive, chicory works just as well.

INGREDIENTS:

1 apple, shaved into thin slices and cut into matchsticks
½ lemon, juice only
½ bulb of fennel, shaved into slices (if you have any fennel fronds, keep these aside for later)
1 head of curly leaf lettuce, washed and torn into pieces
1 head of curly endive, washed and torn into pieces
1 shallot, very finely chopped
4 tbsp extra-virgin olive oil
3 tbsp apple cider vinegar
1 tsp English mustard
1 tbsp honey
sea salt and freshly ground black pepper

METHOD:

Put the apple in a bowl and toss with the lemon juice to stop it turning brown.

In a separate bowl, add the fennel, curly lettuce and endive leaves and scatter over the shallot.

Mix together the oil, apple cider vinegar, mustard, honey, salt and pepper in a small bowl.

Drain the apple and add to the bowl.

Pour the dressing over the salad and toss well to fully coat the leaves. Scatter the salad along the length of a platter. If you have any fennel fronds, throw them on top of the salad and serve immediately.

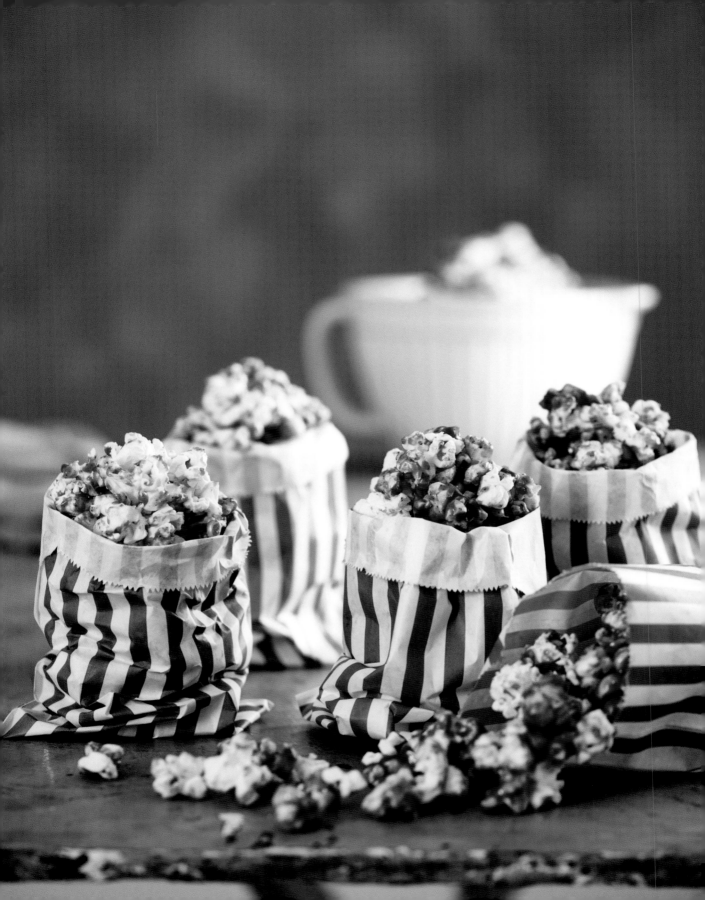

CHAI SPICE AND SEA SALT POPCORN

MAKES
1 large bowl

Movie nights will never be the same again. Hygge your space by grabbing a blanket, lighting some candles and snuggling up with a loved one and this brilliantly easy popcorn that tastes of autumn.

INGREDIENTS:

50g unsalted butter
75g soft light brown sugar
2 tbsp golden syrup
¼ tsp cinnamon
¼ tsp ginger
¼ tsp allspice
1 tbsp vegetable oil
50g corn kernels
sea salt

METHOD:

Line a large baking sheet with greaseproof paper.

Place a pan over a medium heat and melt the butter, sugar, golden syrup and spices. Heat very gently until the sugar has dissolved, then increase the heat and bubble for 4–5 minutes until darkened to a rich caramel colour.

Heat the vegetable oil in a large pan over a medium–high heat. Tip in the corn kernels, cover with a lid and cook until the popping stops (about 5 minutes), shaking the pan frequently throughout.

Pour the syrup over the popcorn and stir until combined. Tip out onto the lined baking tray and spread out in a thin layer. Sprinkle with salt and leave until cooled completely.

HOMEMADE FRUIT GUMS

MAKES
25

Fool the kids into thinking you're giving them sweets, but really, it's all fruit juice.

INGREDIENTS:

4 gelatine leaves
100ml fresh cranberry juice
100ml fresh apple juice
100ml fresh pineapple juice
2 tbsp granulated sugar

EQUIPMENT:

Rectangular tin, approximately 20cm x 20cm lined with grease-proof paper

METHOD:

Soak the gelatine leaves in cold water for a couple of minutes until soft.

Place a pan over a medium heat and heat the fruit juices until on the verge of simmering.

Squeeze the water out of the gelatine leaves and add to the pan, stirring gently until dissolved.

Remove from the heat and pour into the prepared tin. Pop in the fridge to set for at least a 2 hours but preferably overnight.

To create the gummies, carefully slice into squares and lift out of the tin. Sprinkle the sugar onto a board and roll the jellies in the sugar.

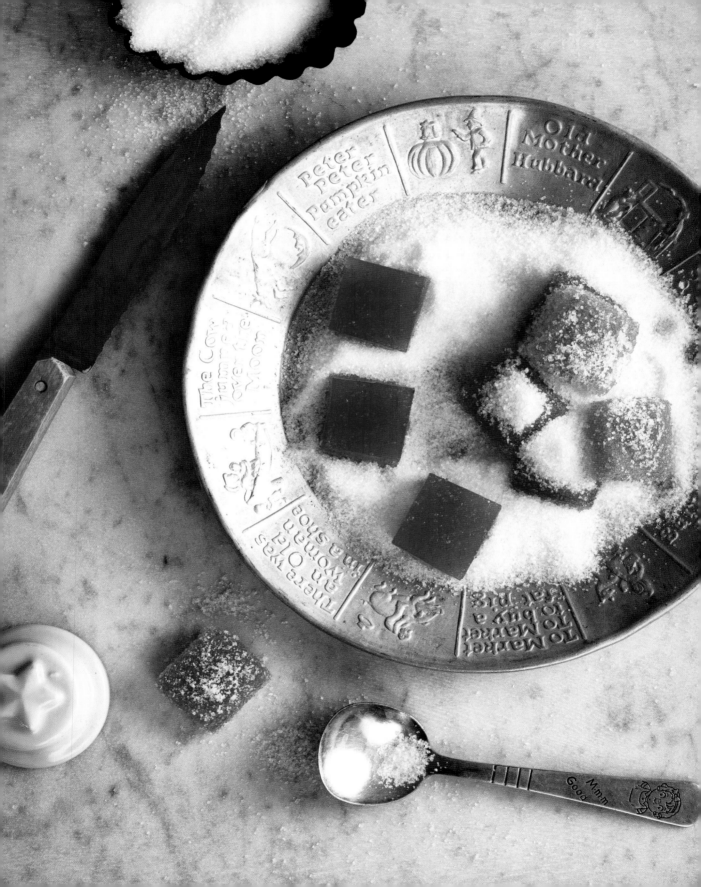

LEMON, LIME AND THYME CURD

MAKES
1 jar

This is gorgeous spread on Mum's Toasted Lemon Drizzle Agave Bread (p 44) and is a key ingredient in Nan's Lemon Mousse (p 177), but it's also perfect on scones as an alternative cream tea (with clotted cream of course), on toast, in lemon meringue pies or straight from the jar.

INGREDIENTS:

zest and juice of 2 unwaxed lemons
zest and juice of 2 unwaxed limes
200g caster sugar
100g unsalted butter
8 sprigs of fresh thyme, leaves stripped from the stalks
5 egg yolks

METHOD:

Put the lemon and lime zests and juices, caster sugar, butter and thyme leaves in a heatproof bowl and gently heat over a bain-marie over a low-medium heat.

In a separate bowl gently whisk the egg yolks and fold into the lemon mixture. Whisk until all of the ingredients are well combined and continue to stir gently over the heat for 10–12 minutes until the mixture is thick and creamy.

Remove the lemon curd from the heat, pour through a sieve over a clean bowl, discarding the thyme leaves. Set aside to cool, stirring occasionally.

Once cooled, spoon the lemon curd into a sterilised jar. It will keep in the fridge for up to 1 month.

HOMEMADE CHOCOLATE SPREAD

MAKES
1 jar

Heavenly on soft fluffy white bread with sliced banana, slathered on hot crumpets, brioche, French toast and crêpes. A treat for your inner child.

INGREDIENTS:

230g skinless, blanched hazelnuts
125g icing sugar
40g good-quality cocoa powder
1 tsp vanilla paste or extract
sea salt

METHOD:

Preheat the oven to 190°C/170°C fan/Gas mark 5.

On a baking sheet, spread out the hazelnuts and bake for 15 minutes until they start to turn golden. Remove from the oven and set aside to cool.

Once cool, transfer the hazelnuts to a blender and pulse for a couple of minutes until they form a smooth oily paste. Then add the remaining ingredients and pulse until smooth.

Transfer to a sterilised jar. It will keep in the fridge for up to 1 month.

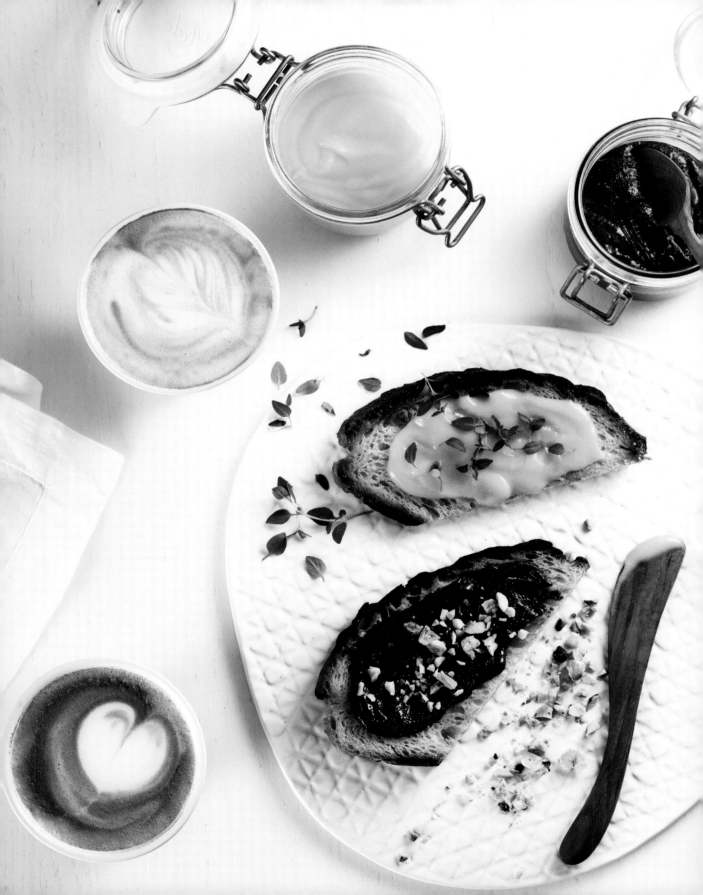

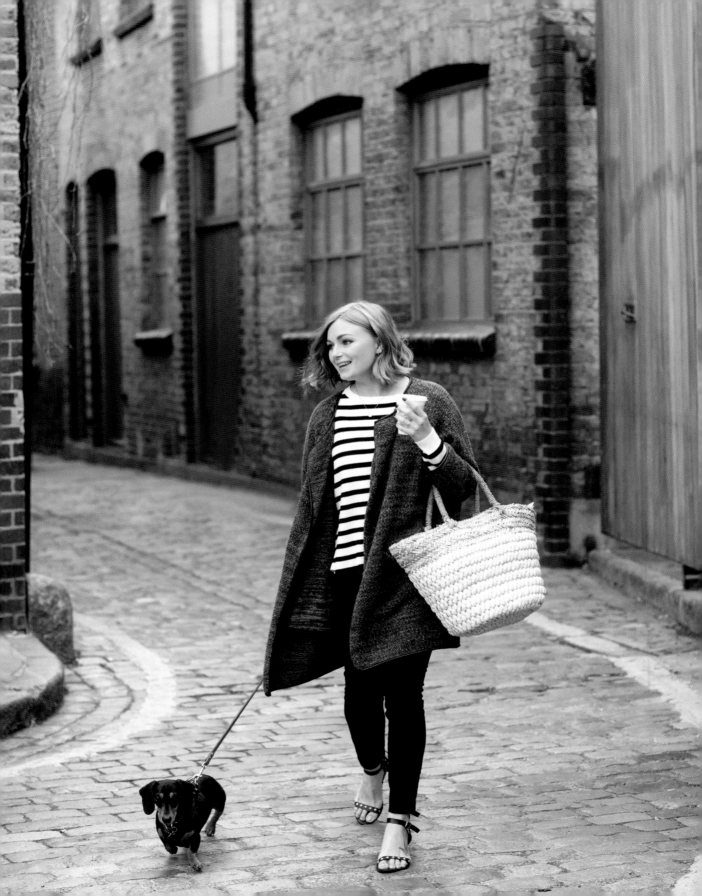

I love making a big picnic in the summer, and have been known to spontaneously take them to the end of the garden to eat by myself! Alternatively, if you have one nearby, visit your local park. Getting out into the open and taking time out for you is such a lovely thing to do. Living in any city, particularly London, is crazy busy and just stopping and sitting on the grass is one of those things that will always, without fail, restore a bit of calm and perspective.

These are the things I like to make for a weekend picnic because they travel well, aren't too messy, and everything can be eaten with your hands. With Darcey leading the way, Mike and I head off to beautiful Richmond Park or Wimbledon Common with a blanket and take some time out.

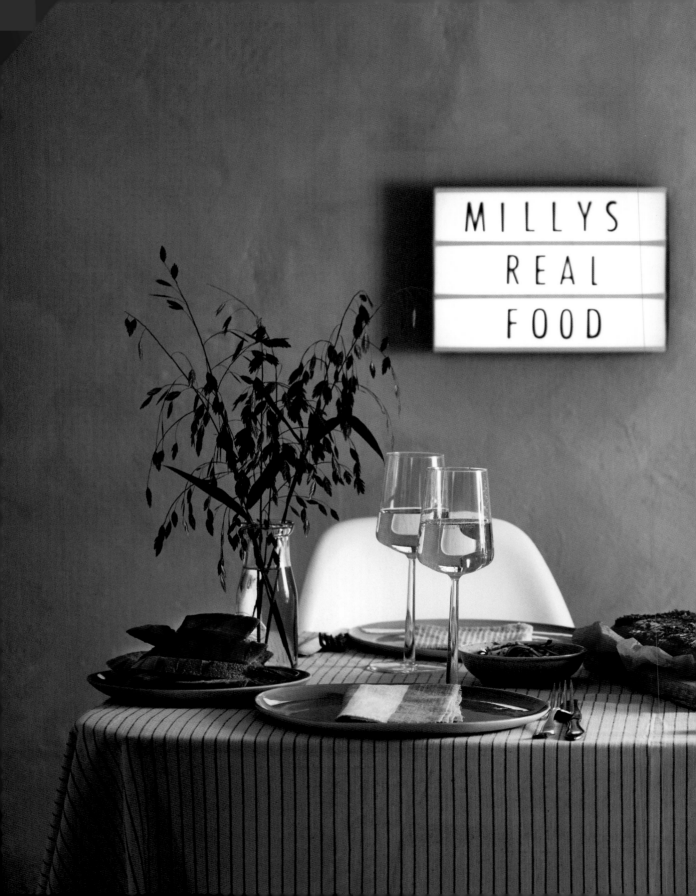

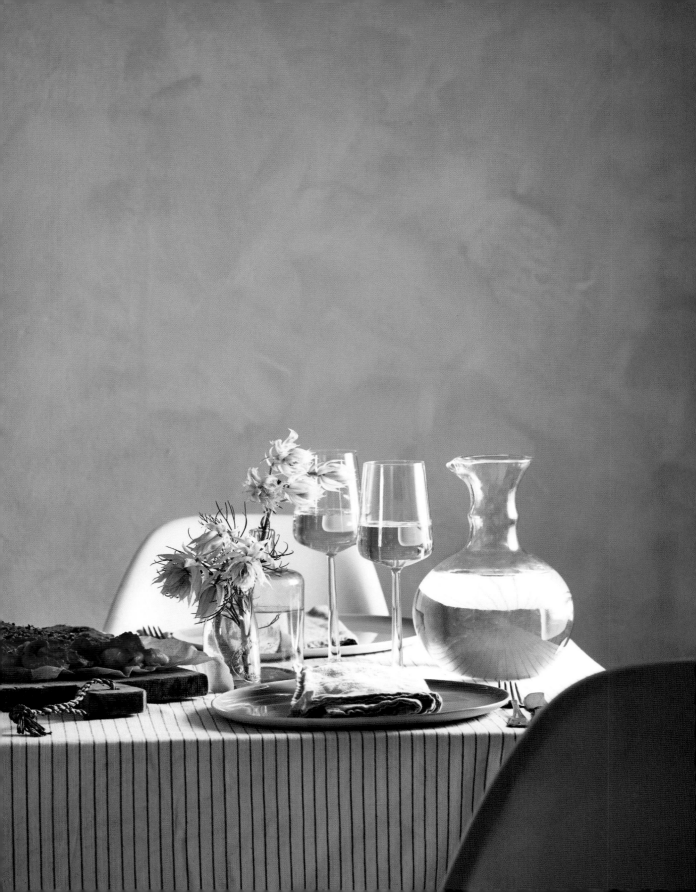

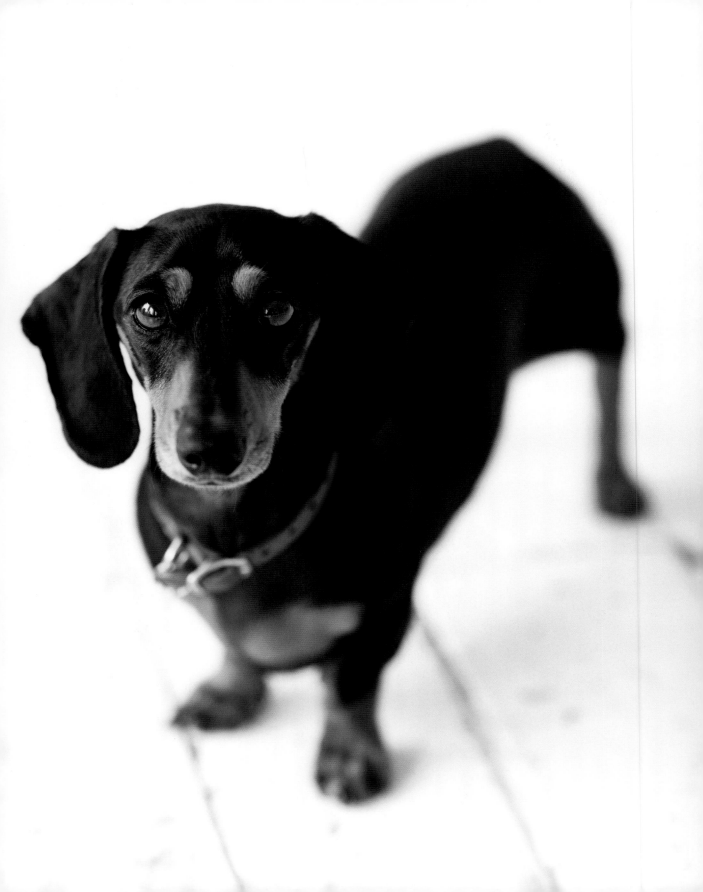

DOG BISCUITS
APPLE AND CHEDDAR BITES

MAKES
over a dozen

In recent years I've made a habit of making dog biscuits for Darcey from scratch. Not only do I have peace of mind that I know exactly what's gone in them, but she absolutely loves them. She watches my every move in the kitchen as I'm making them and seems to know when I'm rustling something up for her!

Like most dogs, Darcey loves cheese but she's also very happy to munch on a wedge of apple, so these biscuits are a combination of two of her favourite things. Darcey doesn't have a wheat allergy, but some dogs do, so these biscuits cater to that. If you're certain your dog is fine with wheat, wholewheat flour is absolutely fine instead of brown rice flour.

Once baked, allow to cool fully before giving one to your pup and will keep in an airtight container for at least 2 weeks.

INGREDIENTS:

1 mug brown rice flour
½ mug shaved apple
¼ mug grated Cheddar
½ mug warm water
1 egg white

EQUIPMENT:

one round cookie cutter

METHOD:

Preheat the oven to 200°C/180°C fan/Gas mark 6.

Mix all the ingredients in a bowl and turn out onto a surface dusted with rice flour. Knead for a few minutes until fully combined and roll out to 1cm thick.

Using a cookie cutter, cut out as many shapes from the dough as possible. Keep balling up the leftover dough and rolling it out until all of it is used.

Place on a lined baking tray, brush with egg white and bake in the oven for 20–25 minutes until golden brown. Allow to cool fully and store in an airtight jar.

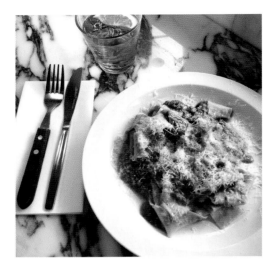

MY
INSTAGRAM
FAVES
@MILLYCOOKBOOK

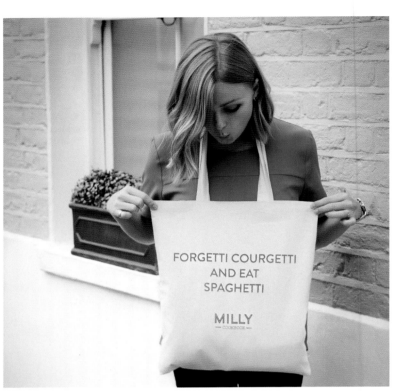

FORGETTI COURGETTI
AND EAT
SPAGHETTI

MILLY

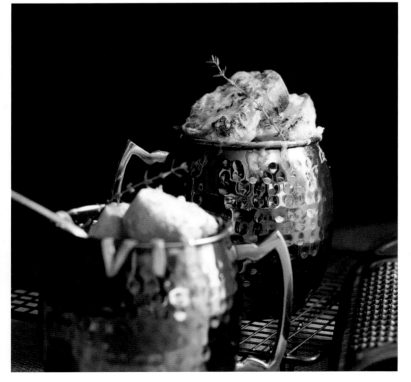

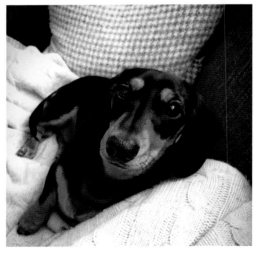

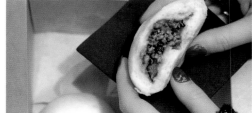

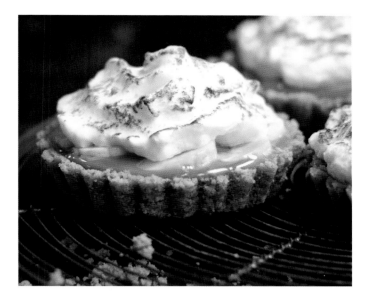

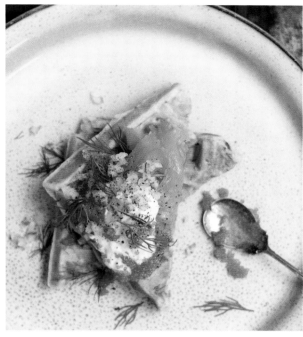

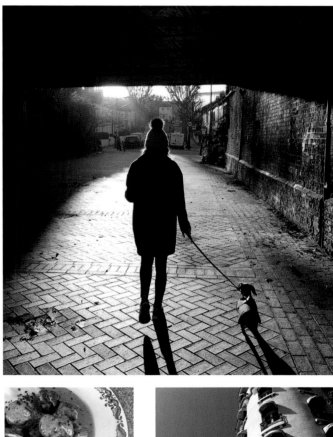

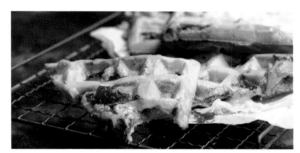

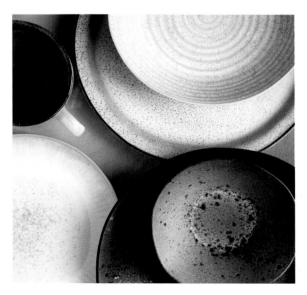

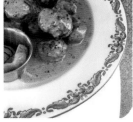

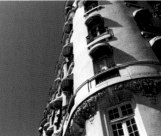

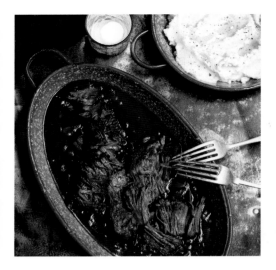

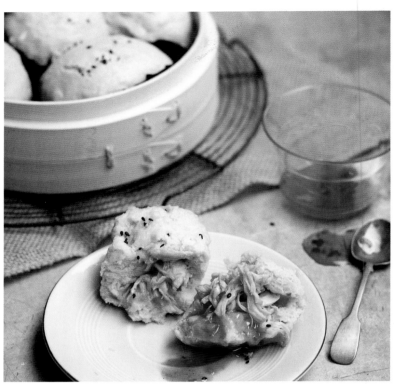

MY
INSTAGRAM
FAVES
@MILLYCOOKBOOK

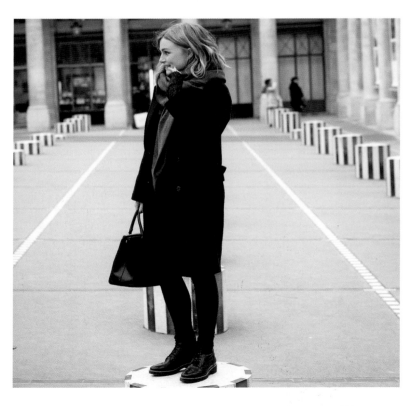

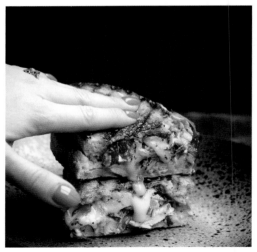

IF YOU PUT AVOCADO IN
YOUR BROWNIE THEN

I CAN'T TRUST YOU

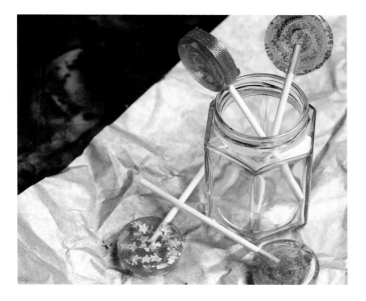
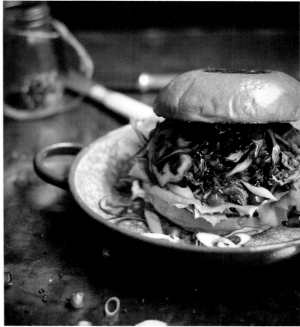
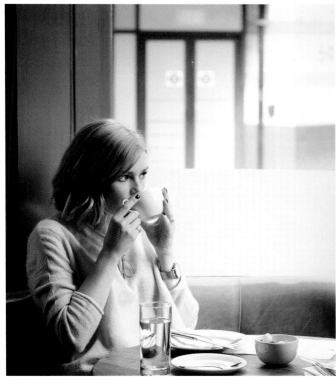
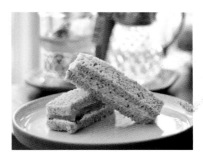
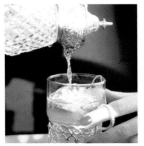
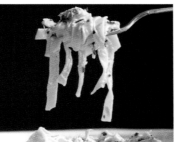
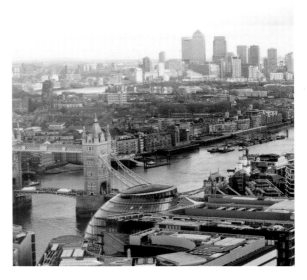

221

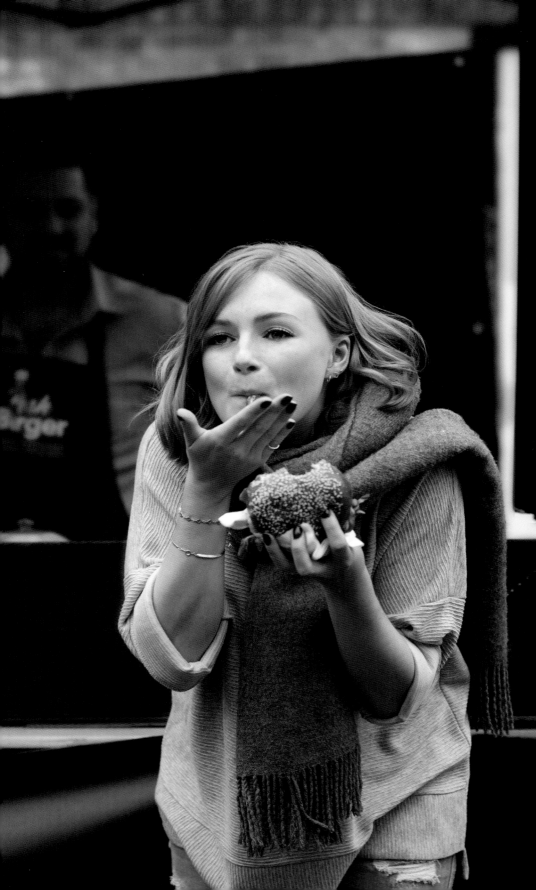

LONDON STREET FOOD AND MARKETS

London's street food scene is undoubtedly at its peak. From cheese toasties to bao buns, the capital is now crammed with stalls serving an array of cheap street eats.

I dream of one day having my very own portable food stall: a clapped-out horse cart transformed into a burger truck. The hatch will rise on the duck-egg blue truck; fairy lights will be draped across the front; white tiles and copper kitchen fixtures will adorn the inside and a pot of herbs will sit on the counter alongside a blackboard reading "Milly's Munchies". Until that day, I rely on the many in town that are absolutely smashing it. There's a lot to choose from out there, but I've been ruthless and picked only my favourite markets which have (in my opinion) the best sellers and heart-stoppingly good food.

Netil Market
South Hackney. Open Saturdays
Head on over to Netil Market, a stone's throw from the nearby and more well-known Broadway Market for the ultimate soft and pillowy pork belly bao buns and Taiwanese fried chicken from Bao London, and the best cheese toastie in town from Morty and Bobs. I highly recommend the M&B Madam and the Mushroom & Truffle Melt.

Venn Street Market
Clapham. Open Saturdays
Down an alley, away from the hustle and bustle of Clapham High Street, lies a hidden market of street food and independent food vendors. As well as fresh produce ranging from baked goods to pâtés, cheese and fish, there's a wide selection of street food such as a hog roast, open sandwiches and dim sum. On a nice day, take your food down to the park, just a two-minute walk away, and enjoy an impromptu picnic. Street food vendors vary each weekend, but if M. Moen & Sons are there with their epic hog roast you're onto a winner.

Street Feast, Dinerama
Shoreditch. Open Thursdays, Fridays and Saturdays
The ultimate foodie's paradise: sample the best street food London has to offer in one trendy arena with ample seating. **Farang:** Fragrant and fresh Thai food. The hot-smoked salmon laska and barbecue chicken satay are a must. **Duck N' Roll:** All things crispy duck. Order the hoisin duck roll and a portion of duck fat fries.

When I'm after top-quality fresh produce, I look no further than London's oldest and largest markets such as **Billingsgate** and **Borough**. But when I'm hankering after a smaller and less frenetic scene, I head to farmers' markets offering homemade cordials, local cheeses and flowers:

Duke of York Square Market
Chelsea. Open Saturdays
Wander down to discover a variety of dim sum stalls, confit duck buns and fish and chips stalls in a beautiful and light-filled setting. Browse and sample mouthwatering charcuterie, cupcakes and cordials followed by a stroll down Kings Road.

Herne Hill Market
Herne Hill. Open Sundays
Browse vintage homeware, nibble on spicy sausages as you meander, and share a cheesy tartiflette and a beer.

Islington Farmers' Market
Islington. Open Sundays
My old stomping ground. Veer off the bustling Upper Street to find yourself in London's first ever farmers' market, set up along an old London street selling homeware, baked goods, street food, flowers, shrubbery and more. There's a little bit of everything here and the greengrocers always have cracking deals.

STOCKHOLM MARKETS AND RESTAURANTS

Stockholm has such a brilliant food scene, but it's quite different to the UK. Street food markets are very popular, but mostly pop up during the summer months. One of the best around is the Hornstulls Marknad, which runs alongside the river and takes place every weekend from April until the end of September. Östermalm is where Mike and I bought our food then we stayed in Stockholm.

Hornstulls Marknad
Hornstul, Södermalm. Open Saturdays and Sundays

A full range of stalls from antique and vintage vendors, arts and crafts and street food stalls. The food available ranges from falafel to burgers, salads to breads and cakes. On a picturesque stretch of southern Stockholm, this is a wonderful place to explore.

Östermalm Saluhall
Östermalmstorg. Open Monday – Saturday

An indoor market full of pretty much everything. Rows upon rows of fresh fish and shellfish; meats and charcuterie; fresh fruit and vegetables; bread, cheeses and chocolates. A fabulous place not only to buy typical Scandinavian crayfish, but to eat it too. Open crayfish sandwiches with crème fraiche, finely chopped red onion, roe and dill is popular for lunch, but be warned – it's very pricey.

Aside from the food markets and summer street food stretch, Stockholm has a number of fantastic restaurants. Cross the river into the trendy southern part of Stockholm and the options are endless. Our favourites are:

BaroBao
Hornsgatan

Stockholm's answer to Bao, London. Order from an illustrated menu and pick from a selection of bao buns, salmon sashimi, beef tartare, slaw and pickles. I must have ordered the Chicken and Pork Belly Bao at least three times.

Bistro Bananas
Skånegatan

A cosy, unpretentious and trendy restaurant. Wood-fired pizzas are the popular dish here, but other Italian mains are available. The Napoletana is, without a doubt, my absolute favourite.

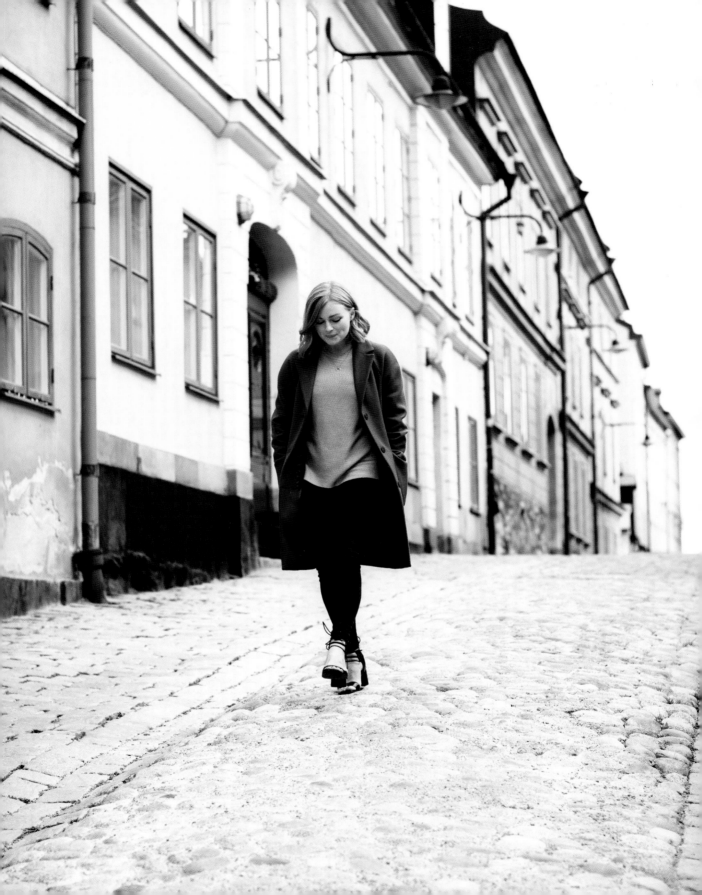

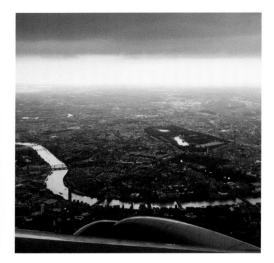

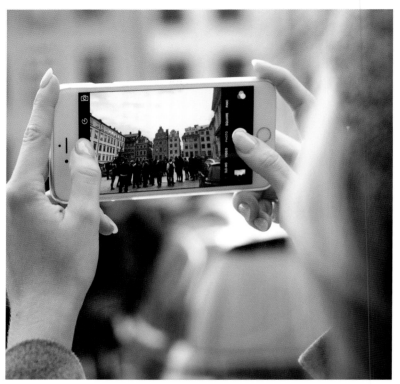

BEHIND
THE SCENES
MILLY'S REAL FOOD

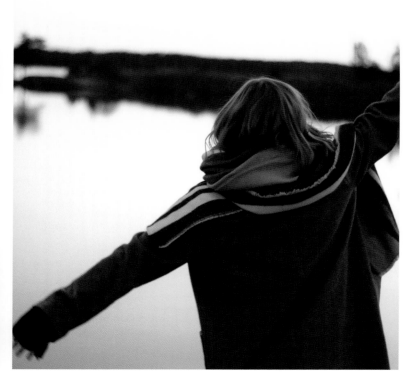

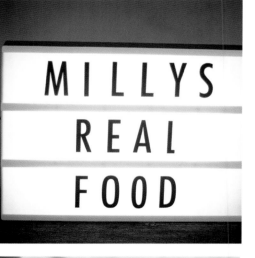

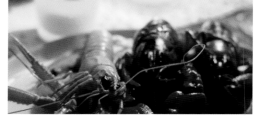

SHOOTING THE BOOK IN STOCKHOLM

Having decided to hire an Airbnb for our ten-night stay in Stockholm, Mike and I find a brilliant apartment on Drottninggatan, a short walk from the centre of town and an even shorter walk from our photographer's studio.

The evening before the shoot starts, Mike, Susanna (our photographer), Sara (a talented Swedish pastry chef and our recipe tester and food stylist) and I head to HarperCollins' Big Book Bonanza event – an opportunity to meet in person the booksellers and the retailers who (hopefully) will be selling *Milly's Real Food!* Then we head off into the night for a delicious group dinner to celebrate our arrival in Stockholm with our publisher, editor and designer.

Makeup artist Katie and hair stylist Kieron fly in the next day to make me more presentable (must learn not to drink wine the night before photoshoots) and we have enormous fun shooting the cover.

The remaining days are all about the food. I like to be very hands-on: Susanna and I pick through her enviable props collection and decide at the beginning of each day which setup we'll use. While she works her magic with the camera and lighting, Sara and I get to work in the kitchen. It takes a few days to sink in that Sara is following my recipes and cooking my food!

At the end of the week Susanna invites us to a crayfish party – a traditional Swedish celebration I've always wanted to go to involving a feast of crayfish, songs and schnapps. Sara has made Västerbottensost, a traditional cheese pie, and Susanna's husband Martin drives until we're just outside of the picturesque town of Trosa.

We arrive at sunset. It's freezing, but beautiful. Maria, Susanna's friend, is hosting at her cabin on the water. It has an outdoor fire and pontoon and I feel like I've dreamt it before. We unload the car, hang up the traditional moon lantern, don crayfish hats, light the fire and set out the food. A guitar is whipped out and the singing starts. We're huddled under blankets, fuzzy from the schnapps and full on crayfish, and the moment feels magical.

Mike and I have the rest of the weekend to explore the city. We head into the Old Town to sightsee in the daytime and head to Rolfs Kök (translating to Rolf's Kitchen, you filthy animal) in the evening; we've already been here twice before. The slow-cooked beef cheek with truffle mashed potato is one of the most delicious things I've ever eaten. The bread is so good that we each eat five rolls every time we go. (We later find out that Susanna shot their first ever cookbook. I can't help but feel it was all meant to be.)

Every morning of the second week of shooting, before we do anything else, the team sits down to coffee, cheese sandwiches and cardamom and cinnamon sticky buns. By now I'm skipping to the studio every day. It dawns on me we're leaving in a few days and for the first time, I'm not so keen on going home.

Come the end of the week, we're amazed at what we've achieved. Susanna's photos exceed every expectation and Sara has taught me so much.

I say a teary farewell to Susanna and Martin, knowing that we'll see them soon. But we're not leaving yet – Sara's taking us out on the town! We drink Margaritas, dance too hard and eat street hotdogs at 3a.m. Eventually Mike and I manage to tear ourselves away and leave the next day to catch our flight home. We spend the whole journey considering moving to Stockholm, but when we come through the door and see Darcey we're glad to be here. We sprawl on the sofa, looking through pictures and cuddling the pup and agree that this was, quite possibly, the best two weeks of our lives.

INDEX

THANK YOU

My apologies. I'm going to gush quite a bit . . .

Friends, family, my girls – you're all ruddy brilliant. Thank you for being super.

Little squid Darcey – you can't read, but I bloody love you, you little sausage. You're the best dog and you've been quite the model.

Richard Jackson – becoming our business partner was a no-brainer. Thank you for your level-headed approach and one-word answers to situations when I wouldn't have even known where to begin. You've been priceless.

Ben Thordycraft – thank you for your tireless evenings, working weekends and 2 a.m. Skype calls. From Day One, you understood brand MILLY and you never cease to amaze us with your endless tech and design talents. You utter dude.

Rachel, Louise and all the team at HQ HarperCollins. Rachel and Louise – you've both been wonderful and I've enjoyed every meeting / drink / dinner we've shared in the UK and Stockholm. Thank you for embracing my pernickety ways and helping me achieve something I never thought was possible.

I owe everything to Lisa Milton at HQ HarperCollins who, from Day One, has had the utmost belief in me and who gave Mike and I the freedom to direct and create this book ourselves. I always had a vision, but Lisa's belief and encouragement made the whole process not only an absolute joy but something that makes us so incredibly proud.

Sara Hultberg – a celebrated chef in your own right, so I am honoured to have you as my food stylist. You've been incredibly gracious and brought my recipes to life.

Susanna Blåvarg – you're one of the most inspiring, kind-hearted and passionate people I've met and from day one you "got me". Thank you for inviting me to shoot at your studio in Stockholm, for making us feel at home in your country, and above all, for your stunning photography.

Mum and Bas – your unconditional love and support knows no bounds. You've been the best parents a girl could ever wish for and I absolutely adore you. Thank you for your constant encouragement, words of wisdom and glasses of wine at 10 a.m. when I've needed to escape the city. You are both my absolute everything, thank you.

Mike – my partner in crime, my soulmate. We've (somehow) created this amazing company and I could not have wished for a better business partner. You're not afraid to call my bullshit and I've inherited a part of your tenacity and sheer determination. I could not, and would not be here without you. Thank you for pushing me to do this and to become what we are. *WE DID IT, POPS.*

And finally, to everyone who has bought my book. My passion and determination to write and create something so close to my heart was uncompromising. Thank you for being a part of the journey and embracing the motto "a little bit of what you fancy does you good". I have poured my soul into writing, cooking, styling and shooting this book and created every page with honesty. I have never been – and never will be – someone who eliminates food groups from their diet to be "healthy", and I hope this book gives you as much joy cooking from it as it has given me embarking on the journey to create it.

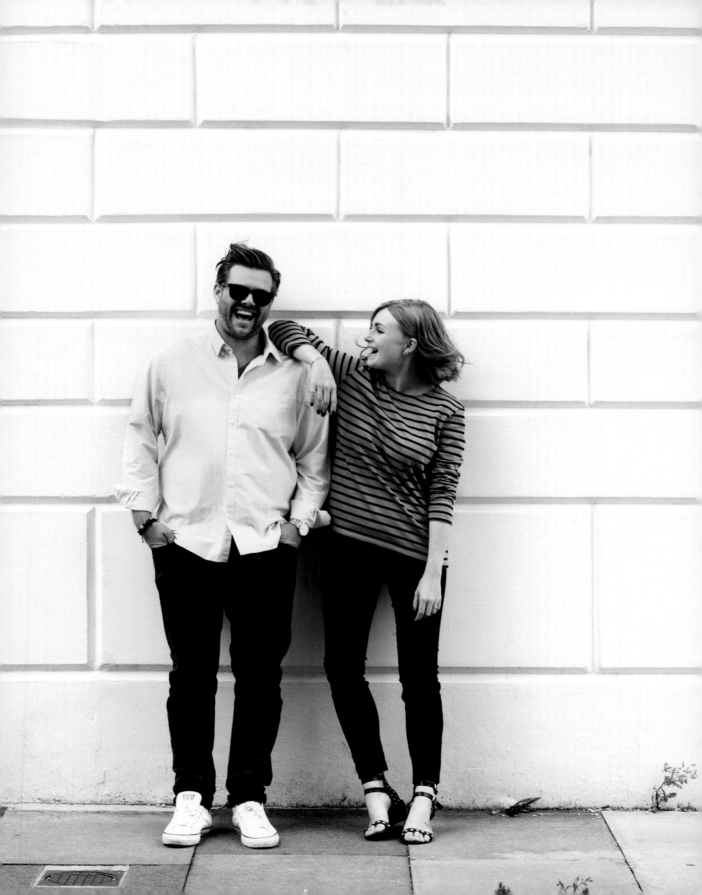

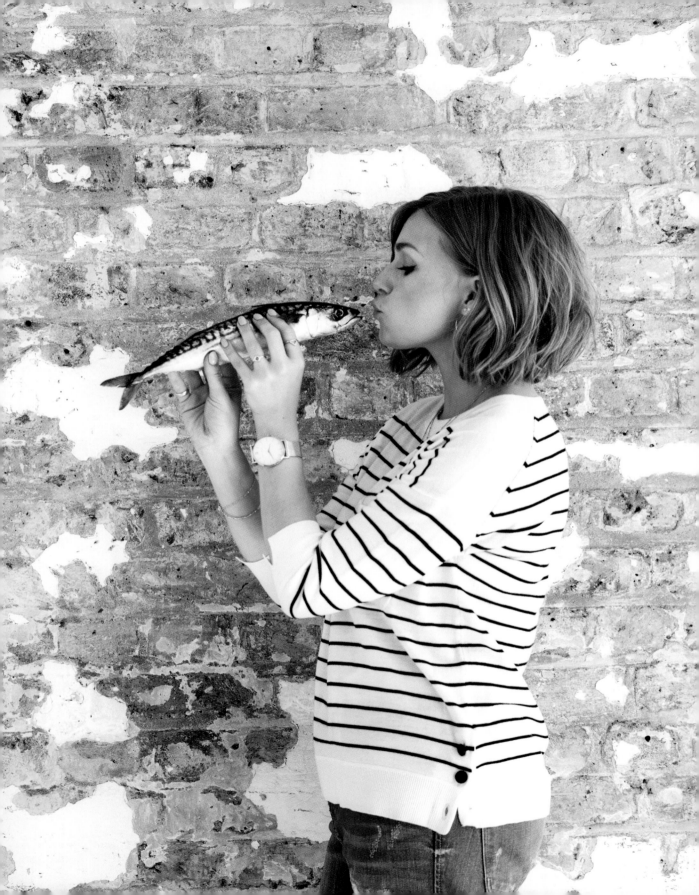